PRAISE FOR
ARE YOU READY FOR A MIRACLE?
... WITH CHIROPRACTIC

"Never before has a book captured the spark of Chiropractic like this one. This book offers insight for every doctor and patient alike. A must read for the skeptic; affirmation for the rest of us."

Dr. Jay M. Holder
Laureate, Albert Schweitzer Prize in Medicine

Are You Ready for a Miracle? ...with Chiropractic

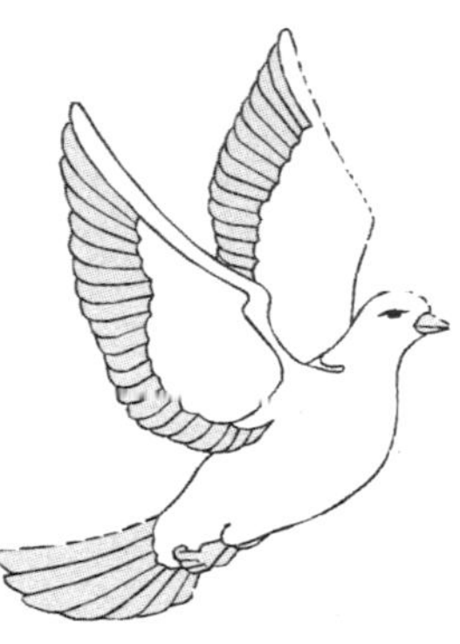

A Practical Guide to Understanding Chiropractic Healing in Everyday Life

CURRENTLY IN PRINT BY ANGELICA EBERLE WAGNER

Secrets of Success :
Excellence ~ The Chosen Path

Are You Ready For a Miracle?
... with Angels

We are currently seeking stories for:

Are You Ready For a Miracle?
... for Children

Are You Ready For a Miracle?
... with Herbs And Vitamins

Are You Ready For a Miracle?
... for Addiction

Are You Ready For a Miracle?
... for The Entrepreneur

Are You Ready for a Miracle?
... for Lovers

Are You Ready for a Miracle? ...with Chiropractic

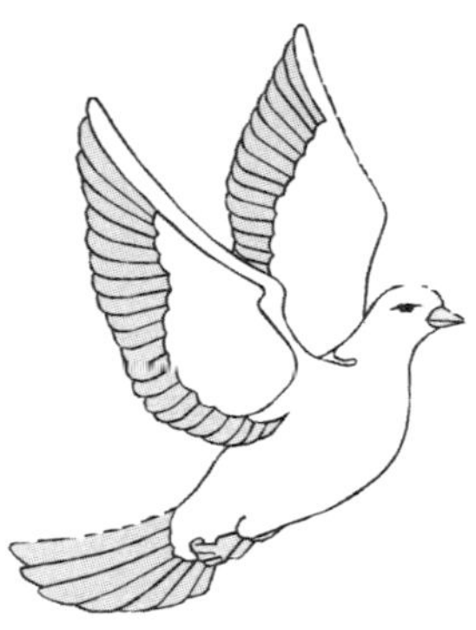

A Practical Guide to Understanding Chiropractic Healing in Everyday Life

By Angelica Eberle Wagner

Miracleworks International Inc.

Canadian Cataloguing in Publication Data

Wagner, Angelica, 1952-
Are you ready for a miracle?—with chiropractic : a practical guide to understanding chiropractic healing in everyday life

ISBN 1-896375-02-2

1. Chiropractic. 2. Chiropractic – Religious aspects. I. Title.

RZ244.W33 1998 615.5'34 C98-931535-5

First Printing April 1999

Cover and book design by
Karen Petherick, Markham, Ontario

Printed and bound in Canada by
Webcom Limited

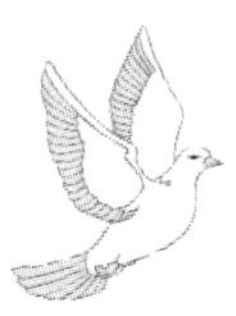

My heartfelt thanks to:

My mother
Christine Eberle Zeeb
healer, advisor, chiropractic advocate

Friends of
"Are You Ready for a Miracle? … with Chiropractic"
The New York Chiropractic Council, Dr. Bob Hoffman, Dr. M. Smatt, Dr.Wm. Remling, Dr. John Di Martini, Dr. Jay Holder and Dr. Marvin Talsky, Dr. J. Gregg, Dr. L. DiRubba, Dr. Brooks, The Canadian Chiropractic Forum, Dr. Marlene Turner, Dr. T. Preston, Dr. B. Moore, Dr. Scott Stevenson.
Thanks also to Dr. Gerry Clum, Dr. Sigafoose, Dr. Nell Williams and Dr. Sid Williams.
Doctors of Chiropractic

I am deeply grateful to all the patients that shared their miracle stories and experiences with me in the writing and creation of this book.

I encourage the healers to continue their work with joy and love. You make a difference. Continue to believe in your healing energy. Live in greater purpose and with greater passion.

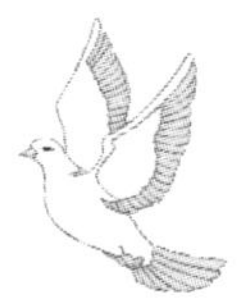

Dear One,

I have written this book just for you. My wish is that you may come to know the magnificence of your own creation. Whatever is hurting your body or your soul, understand that it can be healed. You have been created perfectly in the image and likeness of God. You can release the shackles of whatever infirmity binds you or has bound you.

Today is an instant in your life. You need only to ask for the healing, and you will receive it. Learn to seek the miracles of your birthright, as was intended in the creation and through the great Creator.

The release of the creative life-force energy within you will lead you to greatness. You need nothing. You are enough. You are complete. The great Creator brought you to this time and place to accomplish a great and urgent work. Get up, get on with it, do it now! You are important. I believe in you.

Understand that you are never alone. The angels in their glory were created for you lest you stumble on the smallest stone. Understand above all else how very much you are loved and appreciate the divinity in your soul.

If this book saves only one of you from pain or alters the course of your life through the transformation of your own innate power, it will have been worthwhile in the effect of its energy. The greatness and goodness that lies buried within you needs only to be released one moment at a time for the greatness and goodness of all mankind.

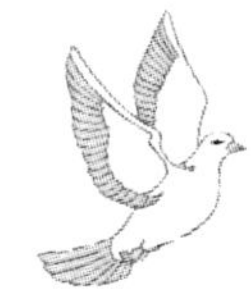

Today is the first day of the rest of your life. Live it well. Energy and time are the blessings of a glorious inheritance. The transformation of the universe lies within your grasp now. Because of the gift and contribution of YOU, the world is better.

Remember, YOU are the miracle!

Angelica

Blessings in Health,
Angelica

Rings and jewels are not gifts, but apologies for gifts. The only gift is a portion of thyself.

~Ralph Waldo Emerson

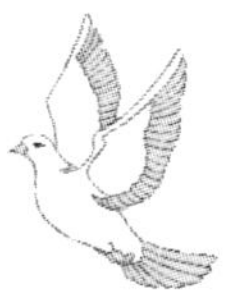

Table of Contents

Part One

Part Two

Part Three

Part One

The Authenticity of Miracles

In the retail world of the 90s the consumer often seeks actively for an authentic product. We search for brand name labels whether that may be in our perfumes, shoes, watches, even jeans. We look for a sign that this product is real. We believe it to be real because there is a label on it showing us that the product was made by this designer or that manufacturer. When we buy jeans, they usually come whole, not with patches on the knees. When we buy new things from a store, we pay for the newness of the product. Sometimes, we even believe that new things are better than old ones and that good products come whole and in one piece. However, God created miracles in our lives to prove that broken, battered, tattered and torn lives have as

Man is born broken; he lives by mending. The grace of God is the glue.

~Eugene O'Neill

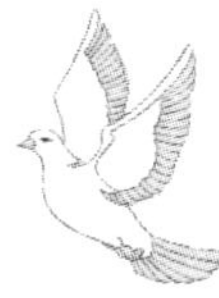

much right to a miracle as those whose lives seem perfect.

By means of miracles, God manifests authenticity in the world. Miracles are signs or sign actions that God has chosen to intervene. These signs show the reality of God as His true self. By means of miracles, God bears witness that He has sent His messengers, the angels to attend and to prove the authenticity of that miracle. This element of divine intervention addresses to humans an urgent message of the will of God. Miracles prove that God is real in our lives and that the work of God is authentic. The angels or healers are sent to attend to the miracle so that His vision for our lives may be unfolded. When we accept miracles as signs and, more important, as actions, the miracles become the label indicating that the product came from God and belongs to us as His children and His heirs.

Everyone thinks of changing Humanity. No one thinks of changing himself.

~Tolstoy

God does not send us miracles to patch up our lives like we put patches on our favorite jeans to make them wearable a little bit longer. He gives us instead a whole new garment, a whole new self. That means we receive a completely new attitude and often a completely new body to authenticate the miracle. God doesn't go just halfway into our lives. He's looking for His own product with His own brand name on it. His own label is authenticated and recognized by the power of love. This is the most complete sign that He has been present. This is the most complete sign of a miracle.

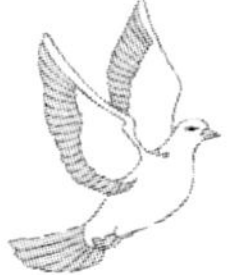

Watch for signs of love around you.

Whether we believe that we deserve this miracle or not is entirely irrelevant. We receive because we already are perfect, and because of who we really are—creations of the divine. That is all we need to recognize and achieve our greatness. No matter what anyone else thinks about you or says to you, you are already great and very deserving of all good things. Begin to live your life that way.

Whatever miracle you need in your life ask for it and expect it.

We become completely new creations when we are the recipients of miracles. The intention of God in our lives is to reveal, authenticate, reform and revolutionize life. Patching you up won't revolutionize who you are. A miracle is sent to transform you. A miracle is sent to create a new being and a new life for each person that the miracle touches. This includes the family and the extended family involved in the miracle.

How else but through a broken heart may love enter in?

~Angelica E. Wagner

Throughout his work on earth, Jesus was known as a healer. His healings were actions that were inspired by the love of those people who needed him and believed. The reason we were created was for deep and never ending love. It is the same reason that we are created to have a deep and never ending love for each other. The greater and deeper the love is that is displayed in actions, the greater and deeper the possibility for life transformation. Have you ever loved anyone deeply enough that they produced a profound change in your life?

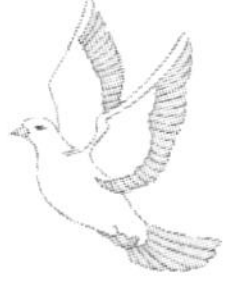

If you have ever loved your work or your life purpose enough to devote yourself totally to it, to be so lost in it that you lose track of time, this is also life transformation.

God always knows exactly what we need and when we need it. If there is a need for a healing in your life, He will heal you. If there is a need for love in your life He will show you a place that you may give it, in order to receive it. One of the miracles of universal law is the law of giving ... as you give so shall you receive. Your need for a miracle will be addressed. Your job is to believe it and ask for it. Keep on asking until it shows up ... often unexpectedly.

Life can only be understood backwards, but it must be lived forwards.

~C.S. Lewis

In the past miracles have happened as an intervention in the paths of destruction that we as humans have chosen for ourselves. In the future miracles will be about complete healing. I have included in this book numerous stories of healings that have already taken place. The shift to healing is a shift that will change the world in its outlook on health and the causes of disease. In the same way it took centuries for scientific facts, flights to the moon and computers to be accepted, the truth on transformation will take time to be accepted. The truth on human healing outside the allopathic model also will take time to be accepted.

The story of love actions shows the true nature of transformation. **In the authenticity of love actions, the label of God's presence is always found.**

Start to look for circumstances and people that show you love in real ways and you will

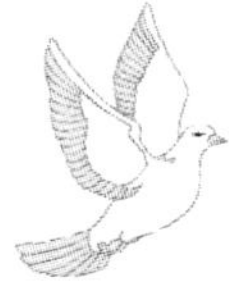

eliminate disease, disaster and tragedy in your life. You will stop the 90-yard dash towards what is not working and begin embracing what does work. You'll start to love your life. Ask yourself these questions:

- In what area of your life do you need a miracle?
- In what area of your life can you create a miracle?
- What greater power is revealed to you because of your pain?
- Are you peaceful about the result?

A feeling of complete peacefulness always accompanies a situation surrounded by love. **This energy creates the miracle.**

Humans are the only creatures who when they lose their way, run faster.

~Jeremiah

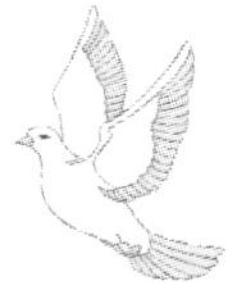

Angel Healers

The problem is more how to still the soul in the midst of its activities.

~Anne Linbergh

C. G. Jung wrote that every patient that falls mentally ill has lost sight of that which basic religions teach: a sense of emotional healing and a deep fulfilling sense of being loved. This is the work of our "earth angels," often appearing as ordinary people in the disguise of healers.

Although I have had the privilege of working with and being in the presence of hundreds of healers, I have not met one who did not feel called to his or her mission. Their purpose is to love and to serve humanity. Their mandate is not just to heal the body, but to endow it with the health of new vitality, energy and life-force spirit. Here in our hearts and our bodies we are most emotionally and physically starved.

The Bible states that it is the will of God to

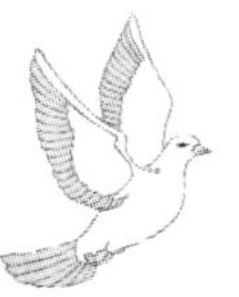

create humans in His own image: all powerful, all creative, all serving, all loving. It takes conscious effort to go against the voices in the world in actualizing the healing powers of nature. It is much easier to believe that the cure for illness is external rather than intrinsic, that we should just take something, swallow something, administer something, cut something rather than unleash our own personal potential in the creation of wellness and wealth in our lives. The power that created the body has the power to heal the body. The aching soul is only a mirror reflection of the body in torment.

The negative ego dwells within us and the darkness of fear surrounds us. The more our internal world is illumined, the more light will be brought to the world. This is easily done by embracing our finest nature. By reaching first for natural means of healing, we are saying to ourselves and to the universe, "I have the power to heal myself and that is where I will begin."

It all begins with a declaration of sovereignty in the body and the soul to regain our independence through natural means and, as a last resort, surgical or pharmacological intervention. It is in claiming our own autonomy that we reclaim the divinity of our souls. The true life-force energy does not come in artificial implants, bottles of pills or even in plasticity of emotion. **It comes from the reality and challenges of being human, of feeling pain, overcoming tragedy and transcending these to joy.**

At the most basic level, angels are sent to

Giving is the secret of a healthy life ... not necessarily money, but whatever a man has; of encouragement, sympathy and understanding.

~John D. Rockerfeller, Jr.

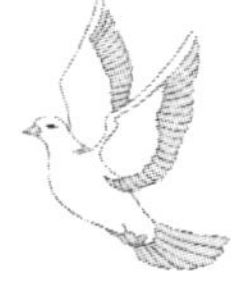

heal the anguish of the human heart, to teach us that we are never alone. Through their presence we can know that we are not rejected, not isolated, not fearful, not in pain. Once this relationship with God through the angels grows and matures in your life, you will experience unlimited power and ease in everything you do … especially as your life purpose is unfolded to you.

Until we experience pain, we do not experience humility. The source of humility then becomes transformed into a source of strength. To go within is not to turn our backs on the world, but to honor the internal essence of our true power, the interrelationship of body, mind, heart, spirit and soul in order to reclaim our own personal sovereignty. Healers, acting as "earth angels," bring us to true purpose by the liberation of our spirits through the liberation of our internal power.

True identity is found going into one's own ground and knowing one's self. One must lose one's life in order to find it.

~Anne Lindbergh

Confronting your darkness causes light to come into your life. In adapting to the new and stronger self, we totally release the negative. When the body systems are free from interference, the body/mind accommodates us to create major change. When our life purpose is free from interference, dreams become our realities.

Inner listening enables us to understand that our first love must be ourselves. The connection to the heart center allows us to feel balance in our lives. As balance occurs, windows of opportunity open. We facilitate our own healing. The chemical changes of the detoxification process allow us to let go of what we earlier

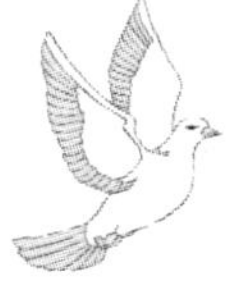

could not release. In discharging this negative energy, we may move into chaos for a while, but it is important to move with this chaos rather than try to control the symptoms.

Discharge is the call to change. It is a massive awakening of the body that change is necessary and imminent. The tension of unresolved feelings accumulate in the body/mind. This tension is resolved through discharge.

Anything that no longer serves your highest good can be discharged from your body, from your life. Any aspect of the self that no longer contributes to healing can be, and should be, let go. The body expresses fever in illness, pushes out blood or pus in infections, causes vomit or diarrhea in intestinal turmoil, fluids in orgasm. The body creates headaches, backaches or illness to tell us that on a cellular level there is trauma. There is chaos. Chaos in our bodies is a good thing and should not be masked by drugs. **Chaos in our bodies reveals the need for change. The cut and paste of surgery does not remove the need for internal change. Surgery resolves chaos only when we have let the situation go on too long. Until the internal tensions are resolved, the body continues to manifest chaos.**

Chaos is essential for meaningful healing and change to take place in our lives. The new-found energy in changing allows us to redirect our lives in harmony with perspectives we have gained. Energy is regenerated in resolution. When we learn to use this internal energy in change, our lives move forward at an unbelievable pace, very

That which hurts most, teaches most.

~ Angelica E. Wagner

I have been schooled to every place and every condition, to be filled and to be hungry, to have abundance and to suffer want. I can do all things in Him who strengthens me.

~Philippians 4:13

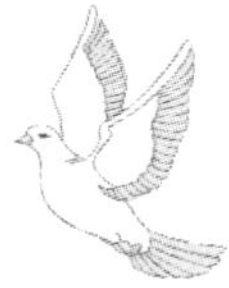

much like a rocket taking off.

The discharge process, like cleaning the closet, is significant. The internal awareness of realignment with the natural order causes the body to show signs of stress. Threat to the physical body is caused by the underlying truth of unresolved chaos in our lives. This transitional stage is enroute to the transformation. Rather than masking it with drugs, we need to feel it. **That means enjoy the process, the pain, stress, chaos, whatever your body is showing you as Truth.**

We must experience the dark threads in the tapestry of our lives in order to appreciate what is golden.

~Angelica E. Wagner

How is your body showing chaos or a need for discharge? How do we respond? Do we apply:

- a band-aid?
- an aspirin or drugs?
- surgery?
- alcohol?
- work?

Or do we embrace the illness, the accident, the failed business deal, the unsuccessful romantic relationship as an urgent call for change?

Then, do we have the courage to move forward in confidence with the changes that are needed to be made in our internal lives so that they show up as healing in our external lives?

Like the gardener pruning the roses in the fall to prepare for the new growth and blossoms of the spring, change must be evident internally before healing takes place externally. **External victory is always preceded by the acceptance of internal Truth.**

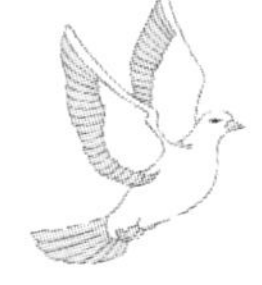

Why Do Miracles Occur?

Miracles occur to reinforce the divine nature of God in our humanity. Miracles are created by God to advance the cause of a humanity that is dying because they believe in tragedy, rather than triumph. In the heart of the anguished soul, lies the truth of the lesson God is sending us for our personal growth. In the very depths of our situations of complete darkness, there is a nugget of truth that solves the dilemma when we just choose to perceive the problem in a different way. Rather than choosing to embrace the darkness and cherish it, the situation becomes a miracle when we embrace the light that is always at the core of the miracle, and learn to cherish that light instead.

God has not called us to see through each other, but to see each other through.

–Galatians 6:2

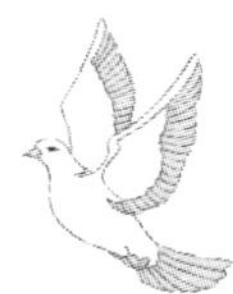

When Do Miracles Occur?

When an inner situation is not made conscious, it appears on the outside as fate.

~C.G. Jung

In waiting for a miracle to occur, sometimes strange events happen that give us clues that a miracle is on it's way. When you need a miracle, all you need to do is ask for one and it will show up when it is meant to occur. There are no unreasonable miracles, only unreasonable time frames for expectation of the miracle to occur. Actually anyone can have a miracle, if you believe that you deserve one.

The miracle is preceded by a syncronicity of events that will occur surrounding your request. Unfamiliar people will come into your life to take your hand to lift you higher. They will help you more than you could ever help yourself with your own powers. If you allow yourself to follow their advice, your miracles will occur effortlessly.

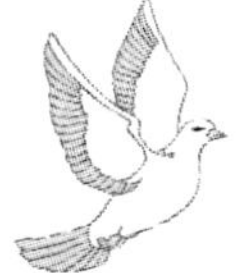

Sometimes miracles are also preceded by dreams, intuitions or events that are in direct contradiction with the current situation.

A miracle is usually preceded by a sign, a sign-action, or a wonder of nature. A sign of your request begins slowly at first, like small amounts of money when you need it, or a small healing in your body before complete healing occurs. A sign-action is always a sign of love that requests nothing in return. Sometimes love will come in an unexpected place from an unexpected source at the same time that you need love.

A wonder is a sign of nature that is sent by God to show you that you are not alone and that the situation is under control. In the area of wonders, I have had reports of northern lights when they were not expected, raccoons in the middle of the city on train tracks, herds of elk on the front steps of a hotel waiting for the recipient, falling stars made visible only to the one who needed the miracle. These are just a few examples of wonders occurring prior to miracles.

When you are certain that you are willing to surrender to the worst happening in the consequences of your situation, there is generally a sign, a sign-action or a wonder that occurs when a miracle is ready to make itself known to you.

When you feel a complete sense of peacefulness and resolution in the situation, the miracle will make itself known to you. This is the essence of the God source that is in all of us.

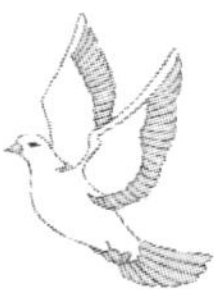

There will be a counterforce of energies that creates the miracle. As more people begin to talk about miracles, more miracles will occur in complete harmony with God's great purpose in our lives. Correction and healing in our bodies and our souls will result from the shift in thinking that all things are accomplished with love. The circle of love goes on and on connecting our humanity, joining one to another.

Heaven is the awareness of perfect unity within the universe in our lives, here and now.

Man looks at outward appearances. God looks at the heart.

~1 Samuel 16:7

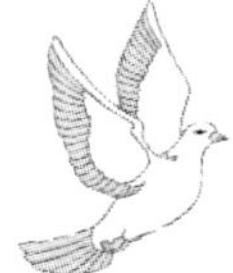

The Need for Miracles

All people smile in the same language.

~Proverbs 15:13

Miracles express God's intention of wholeness for society. It is this intervention of God in our lives that restores, heals and liberates humans to a place of dignity and power. The message of the miracle is that we are powerful beyond measure. Are we aware of our own powers? Do we act on them?

As we begin to acknowledge miracles in our lives, we begin to acknowledge being stuck in our lives, remaining in any state that is restricting, constricting or limiting in any way. However, when we are clear about who we are, the energy that is around us and in us flows freely. We experience no strain. A feeling of happiness or peacefulness accompanies miracles.

When we resist the energy of the universe or

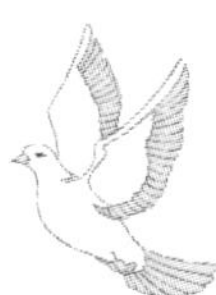

of our soul pointing the way to greatness in our lives, we experience a shaky, out-of-control feeling. We believe these shaky feelings are bad for us. They scare us. However, truth is expressed in accepting these shaky feelings, feelings of insecurity or vulnerability, as a sign that we are on the right track. **As we learn to embrace uncertainty and move toward it with with trust, miracles unfold in our lives**.

Does it mean that travesties or tragedies are placed in our path in order to illuminate our power rather than to diminish it? Isn't that our greatest fear?

Earth has no sorrow that Heaven cannot heal.

~Thomas Moore

In his 1994 inaugural speech, Nelson Mandela summed this up very well using words from Marianne Williamson in "A Return to Love."

Our deepest fear is not that we are inadequate.
Our deepest fear is that we are powerful
beyond measure.
It is our light, not our darkness that most
frightens us.
We ask ourselves, who am I to be brilliant,
gorgeous, talented, or fabulous?
Actually, who are you not to be?
You are a child of God.
Your playing small doesn't serve the world.
There is nothing enlightened about shrinking so
that other people won't feel insecure around
you.
We are all meant to shine, as children do.
We were born to make manifest the glory of
God that is within us.

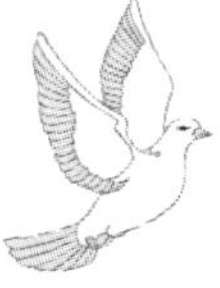

It is not just in some of us; **it's in everyone**.
And as we let our own light shine, we
unconsciously give other people permission
to do the same.
As we're liberated from our own fear,
Our presence automatically liberates others.

Fear is one of the insidious and powerful prisoners of mankind. It is the feeling of impending doom or disaster in whatever we undertake that imprisons us. Like the Rock of Alcatraz, we become impenetrable, until the walls of doubt come cascading and crumbling around us. Perhaps the greatest psychological debilitator of all time is the fear of success. We choose to be imprisoned by failure, by pain, by the frailties of our bodies, and repeat that imprisonment rather than to move out of our comfort zones to try something new, in order to meet and greet success as we would an old friend.

But the very hairs of your head are all numbered.

~Matthew 10:30

People stay locked in careers they should not be in, locked in partnerships they should not be in, locked in marriages they should not be in, in order to remain in the stability of that state. To be out of control, to be out of balance, to be out of public expectation causes such feelings as insecurity, guilt, physical harm, disease or death. When feelings of fear are ignored or defended against, they actually create a magnetism that draws the occurrence of the feared result into actuality. "Whatever you think about, you bring about." Has that ever happened to you? Has what you feared greatly and deeply come upon you?

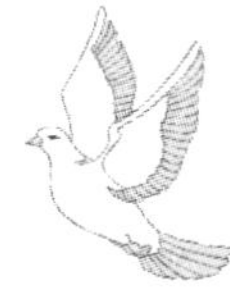

Recognition of the need for a miracle in your life begins by acknowledging that a state of depression, dysfunction or disease is a sign of the need for change, followed by embracing all those frightening emotions that take us in the direction of that change and living our lives by "going with the flow"—or being in the flow rather than using the change and the scary feelings that we all feel as reasons for remaining in the "stuck place."

It is reclaiming our own power and the intensity and fullness of that power that should be directing us, rather than remaining in a state of being half-comatose in our lifestyle and in our decisions. By choosing not to live life, take risks, do something new, have fun, we live—actually live—half-deaths. Life gives us the tragedies to wake us up to the possibilities of enjoying each day, each hour, each minute, each second.

Seek and you will find it. What is unsought will also go undetected.

~Sophocles

So what's stopping you from taking the risks you need to take in order to be fully alive? Why are you staying stuck? Is it easier to be stuck than to overcome what's really going on?

We tend to live life as though we are hooked up to the intravenous bottle of doubt and, whenever a miracle arrives on our doorstep, we take another dose of doubt, Demerol, or some other current drug of numbness in order to remain in the old state. When we recognize fullness, freshness and reality of living the miracles in life with all its glory and power, this is so frightening that this thought keeps us addicted to half-deaths and half-truths. **What are you denying about yourself that keeps coming up?**

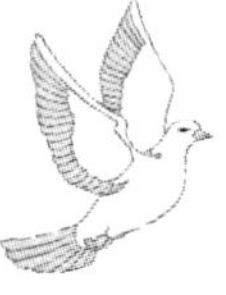

If you choose not to seek the truth of your own greatness, you will continue in stuck patterns that lead nowhere. But you can be delivered from states of darkness by seeking the light of your own deliverance and embracing an alternative way. Choose to seek a change in your life. In the final analysis, it's the only way, as it embraces the truth that your body craves and needs for optimum health.

Ask yourself:

- What is withholding the flow of energy and happiness in your life?
- To acknowledge your drug of choice and forgive yourself for taking it. Whatever that is ... we all have addictions.
- To give recognition and acknowledgment to your fears, rather than dismissing them.
- To name ten major life goals and ten major accompanying fears that are imprisoning you.

Break Free!

Finding fault is like washing windows. The dirt is always on the other side.

~Psalms

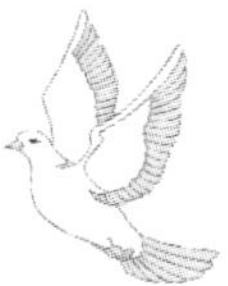

Part Two

The Miracle of Chiropractic

Chiropractic is a unique and very specific science. It deals with the structures of the body, primarily the spine and spinal nerve systems, and the relationship between the proper alignment of those structures and bodily functions. It is a science firmly grounded in anatomy, physiology, neurology and biomechanics. Unlike other approaches to healing, Chiropractic seeks to maximize the inherent recuperative powers of the human body and by acting to realign structural elements of the spine through the process of the Chiropractic adjustment, to remove blockages to proper function.

Chiropractic defines improper spinal alignment as the "subluxation complex." This condition, which is very common, involves

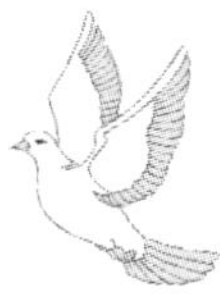

everything from muscle and soft-tissue strains to severe impingements on spinal nerves because of out-of-place vertebrae causing a vast array of symptoms and conditions. The Chiropractic adjustment is a safe, carefully planned clinical intervention that is delivered more than a million times each working day in the United States alone. Chiropractic is a natural approach to health and health care and offers the consumer an effective, drug-free, non-surgical alternative for a wide range of conditions.

The Chiropractic profession is the second largest primary care health care profession in the world and the fastest growing. In the U.S., there are more than 55,000 licensed Doctors of Chiropractic, with 11,000 students currently enrolled in professional studies. Doctors of Chiropractic must complete a rigorous program of four years of full-time, resident postgraduate instruction and then pass a series of difficult examinations at both a national and state level before they are granted a license to practice. All 50 states officially license Doctors of Chiropractic as portal-of-entry provides, to which any citizen can go for care without prescription or referral from any other provider.

Chiropractic is also recognized by dozens of nations throughout the world, from Canada to New Zealand, and the profession is growing rapidly throughout the world, largely because of its effectiveness in dealing with so many conditions on a highly cost-effective basis. This ability is particularly vital in less affluent countries that do not have massive amounts of

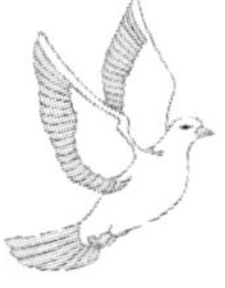

resources to spend on expensive drug and surgery-based conventional medical treatments, especially when an effective substitute approach is available through Chiropractic.

In our contemporary age, when individuals are seeking to take control of their own personal health and health care decisions, Chiropractic is very much in tune with the values and priorities of a society seeking a natural, safe and effective choice in health care services. If you read the popular press or watch television, you consistently see stories about the end of the drug era as bacteria and virus strains are emerging, immune to the drugs and treatments that contained them in the past. You also see constant reporting of a popular quest for better health through diet, exercise, environments that are free from toxic chemicals, and ways that are ergonomically appropriate.

At the same time, health challenges are changing with new conditions that result from career obligations such as carpel tunnel syndrome that is said to result from continual computer data entry work. Chiropractic offers a powerful intervention that seeks to maximize the benefits of the wellness lifestyle, as well as a means to address a vast array of conditions that are painful, costly and often difficult to care for.

In 1995 the Chiropractic profession celebrated 100 years of existence as a separate and distinct science and profession. During that 100 years, Chiropractic grew in spite of intense anti-competitive pressures from critics and competitors in the academic and commercial

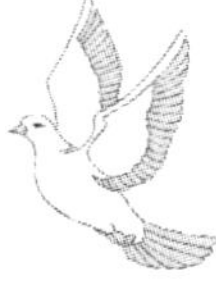

health-care marketplaces. There is no doubt, however, that the sound, effective nature of Chiropractic care has proved the utility of this still emerging science. In the next century, scientific and clinical research will continue to unlock the mysteries of how Chiropractic works, and how it can be made more effective. Doctors of Chiropractic will continue to provide safe, effective clinical care to a growing number of millions throughout the world, applying their unique skills and science with careful clinical attention, human compassion and concern.

Dr. James Gregg
Chairman of the Board
International Chiropractic Association

Other people don't create your spirit, they only reveal it.

~Brandt

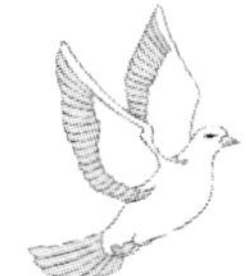

Introduction

Since all individuals are responsible for their own actions and cause their own effects, optimism is a choice.

~Dennis Waitley

Are You Ready for a Miracle? ... with Chiropractic was written by the patients of Chiropractic care for the thousands of Doctors of Chiropractic that are the unsung heroes of healing. Although there are millions of cases of complete healing through Chiropractic care, Doctors of Chiropractic are still regarded as mysterious and somewhat radical in both their techniques and their integrity as healers. There is still a dark cloud of suspicion over the profession and a dread of witchcraft. Nothing could be further from the Truth. It is also a known fact that until as late as 1975 chiropractors were jailed for practicing the healing art of Chiropractic.

Chiropractic is not only a science, philosophy and art of healing; it also requires that the head,

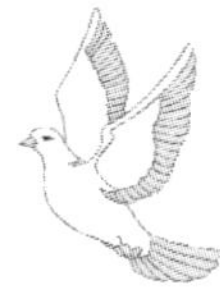

heart, and hands of the Chiropractor be completely in tune with this art. The knowledge of the adjustment is learned through many years of study and practice. The loving energy of the healer through the skill of his or her hands releases the places in the body that are restricted due to nerve interference.

In healing, energy is transmitted from the head, heart and hands of the healer through the patient's body needing the care. Healing occurs because the Doctor of Chiropractic knows where the body is not in harmony with itself, and releases this interference through the power of the adjustment. In Chiropractic circles it is called "the power of the innate." This innate force within the body knows how to conquer disease. Our bodies do know how to heal ourselves.

To every thing there is a season, and a time to every purpose under heaven.

~Ecclesiastes 3:1

This book gives testimonies from patients who have received Chiropractic care. The book is in actuality a very large thank-you note from all those who are grateful to have the health that the allopathic or medical model could not provide for them in their circumstance.

This book presents evidence that double blind studies, rigorous documentation or years of science do not hold all the answers to the cures of disease. It began with my own struggles with health. After a freak car accident many years ago, I was left unable to walk for several weeks. I explored all avenues of general medical procedures with no improvement and finally turned to Chiropractic care as a last resort.

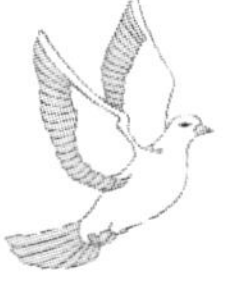

To my amazement, I was healed. It was a miracle!

Since then, with several sports injuries later, Chiropractic has become a regular part of my health care and the health care of my family. We could not lead active lives without this natural way of keeping well.

It has taken several years to collect the miracle stories that follow. Chiropractors are reticent to talk about their own miracles. In many areas of North America, the skill of their care and their healing abilitites are still not recognised and are blatantly dismissed as quackery. Although hundreds of stories have been submitted, we could not choose them all. In gratitude we included the most dramatic ones to make the point that natural health care works. If these stories give hope or encouragement to even one person, these efforts will have been worthwhile

If you have not yet explored the benefits of natural health care through Chiropractic, we hope that these stories will inspire and encourage you to lead your life differently. Before surgical intervention becomes necessary, look at the alternatives. Our bodies were created as the divine vessels that take care of our souls. We were created with the divine capacity to heal ourselves.

Hypocrites said, "Look well to the spine for the cause of disease." If the father of medicine was examining the nervous system for the solutions of disease in the first century, why are

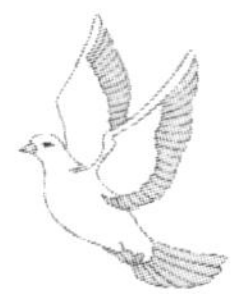

we not also seeking the answers there now?

These stories resonate with the love of the doctors for each patient and with the love of the patients for their healers. Thank you to all who contributed from their hearts and their experiences to write this book with me.

Chiropractic Stories

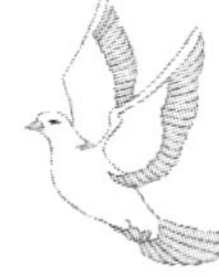

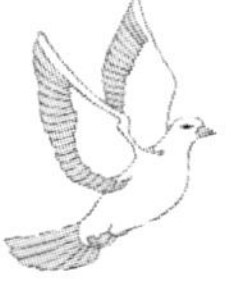

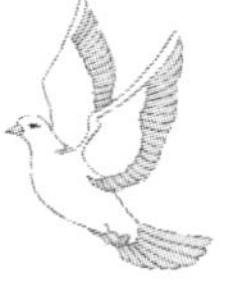

A MIRACLE OF NATURE

• *Mrs. Mamie Ruth Poston*

I started to have sharp pains in my back. The pain would move up and down my spine and would cut my breath off. In a short time the pain went into my legs. My legs started to swell, draw and feel heavy. I went to a specialist who said my kidneys were bad. I was put in the hospital and then told I had pulled muscles and an infection. I was given shots every four hours for pain and pills for the infection. I was put in traction for one week.

After this my legs got so heavy and numb I couldn't use them and would have to be carried everywhere. The doctors then said they didn't know what was wrong with me. I left the hospital and returned home with my legs paralyzed and I had no feeling from the waist down. It was a very depressing thing to be helpless and have to depend on others to move me and help me, especially with a child and husband that I needed to look after.

While waiting for my appointment at Duke Hospital, my mother asked me to try a chiropractor because she knew people who had been helped. I will never forget what followed!

I went to the chiropractor on Saturday, carried in a wheel chair by my husband. The chiropractor made an X-ray of my spine and showed us how an old injury was causing the nerves not to work properly. He gave me my

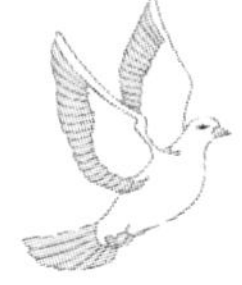

first adjustment. On Sunday I got another adjustment. On Monday morning I could move my legs off the bed. This was the first time in two weeks that I was able to move them by myself. I cried and praised God.

That morning my mother took me to the chiropractor. He adjusted me again and it felt like new life came into my legs. I got up off the adjusting table myself and walked. I walked all around the chiropractor's office and my mother joined me in crying for joy.

Words can never say how I thanked God, the chiropractor and Chiropractic for giving me the strength to walk again! I now have a body without pain. Nature truly is wonderful. Pills could never do it.

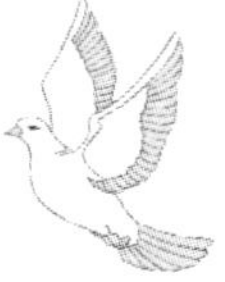

ALL IN THE FAMILY • *Mrs. Ruby Smith*

Forty-five years ago my husband got hurt at work and broke his back. He was in the hospital for some time and couldn't move even a toe. He could only move his hands, arms and his head from side to side.

When he was released to come home, they didn't know if he would ever work again. Our family doctor said he didn't like to operate on the back. He advised my husband to contact a chiropractor. He said he would sign the compensation documents to pay for Chiropractic treatments. It was cheaper for compensation to pay a chiropractor than it was to have a back operation in those days. Since then my husband was healed and has danced a lot.

My six-year-old daughter had a mastoid which left her deaf. We took her to all the ear, eye, nose and throat specialists that we could; none could help her.

Her teacher said she couldn't get through to her year at school because she could not hear. The chiropractor wanted to know why Joan didn't answer him. My husband said, "Oh! I forgot to tell you she is deaf. She has to see you and read your lips." The chiropractor had never treated deafness but wanted to adjust her. We were happy to try anything. After four treatments we noticed a difference. She actually heard me. He adjusted her and she can hear perfectly now.

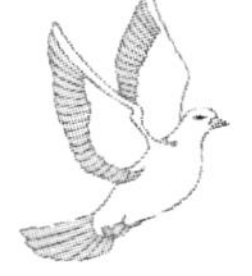

I also have rheumatoid arthritis, osteoarthritis and rheumatism in nerves and muscles. I am very thankful to have Chiropractic doctors available that can help keep me going. I drive my car and still do a lot of things. At 80 years of age, I'm lucky!

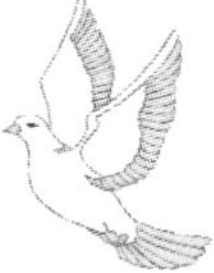

ALLERGIES • *The Patterson Family*

Dear Dr. Larry,

We would like to thank you for what you have done for Denis. As you already know when Denis was one month old he was admitted to Primary Children's Hospital. Denis was first admitted for an allergy to milk and too much acid in his body. As soon as Denis was admitted he started to dehydrate. His stool was runny as water, his face and his body was discolored. He was thin and very sick. The hospital turned out to be a very long and costly visit. They did test after test and put Denis through pure hell for fifty-nine days from October 7, 1981, through December 6, 1981.

First of all, while Denis was in the hospital, he became malnourished. Denis weighed six pounds and his twin brother Danny, at three months old, weighed 11.5 pounds. At birth Denis was 5 lb. 13 ounces and Danny weighed 4 lb. 13 ounces. When Denis was finally released on December 6, we still didn't know what caused his problems and neither did the doctors.

Well, we finally got Denis home, and he seemed to be doing all right. When we had him home for about three weeks, he started having seizures and getting sick all over again. He was admitted to Primary Children's Hospital on January 8. They did more tests and kept Denis for six days. We still did not find out what caused Denis to have seizures. One of the

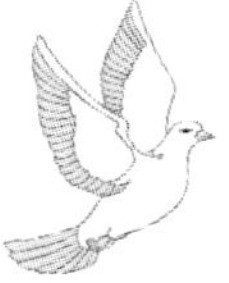

doctors told us that Denis had both mental and physical developmental delays. These would put Denis about three months behind his twin brother Danny.

We would like to tell you that after we brought Denis to you we came to find out that Denis did not have physical and mental developmental delays at all, but was just too weak and sick to act like a normal, healthy boy. All the problems Denis had were because of his spine.

When we first brought Denis to your office at the age of one and a half years, he was still on projestimil and could not eat solids. We were told he might get sick all over again according to the medical doctors. He was still underweight when we brought him to you. Denis could not walk; he could hardly crawl. He never played much, never smiled or laughed, or did any of the things that his twin brother was doing. He was very lazy and inactive, we thought, for a boy his age.

On Denis's first visit to you, you took him off the projestimil and put him on goat's milk, which dropped our milk bill for Denis from $120 a month to $18 a month. With his weekly treatment with you he started to slowly catch up both mentally and physically with Danny. His activity was a lot better. He started eating solids. He started walking and eating with a spoon. He started to play, laugh and smile, like a normal, happy little baby. He caught up developmentally and is now a very happy little boy.

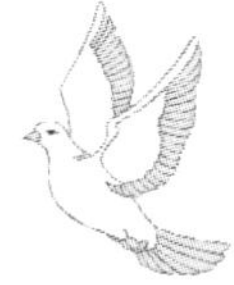

Dr. Larry, we could not begin to express our gratitude and feelings in a letter, but we hope you understand how it feels to have our son back. Dr. Larry, you did what took specialists at Primary Children's Hospital over 159 days of hospitalization and $60,000 of medical bills to try and find out Denis's problem. They still failed. You found and corrected, without pain or drugs, what seemed to us overnight, a situation we did not know how to fix.

We think your treatments of Chiropractic care are terrific. If more people could see this and realize the body's self healing abilities with Chiropractic care, there would not be any more illness. We thank you, Dr. Larry, from the bottom of our hearts. We hope you will share this letter with other people so that they, too, can see what Chiropractic care can do!

ANTIBIOTIC OVERDOSE • *Kim Cheeseman*

With a birth of a child, a parent only wants the very best for that child with health and their future. In some cases, as in mine, that can't always be achieved.

Lauren's life has been a constant struggle for health and well-being. It was at the early age of eight weeks that a severe gastrointestinal infection hit, with a lengthy recovery of eight weeks and many antibiotics. Constant colds and viral infections seemed to be the norm. At one year it was potentially fatal, viral encephalitis that almost cost our precious little girl her life. The fight continued with over 14 months of follow-up that included CT scans, brain scan, anti-convulsants and more antibiotics. By the age of two and a half, allergies and asthma had set in. The prescribed drugs of choice consisted of two different inhalers, eye drops and cortisone nose spray. How much more could her little body endure? After six months of this regimen and a bout of pneumonia, I knew as a mother I couldn't bear putting any more rounds of antibiotics into my daughter's body.

It was at this time that Chiropractic was suggested, but what could Chiropractic possibly do for her? How could it help with total health care? I had to try.

After several weeks of adjustments, I began to notice a change in Lauren. Her constantly runny nose was now dry. After three months of constant care, she no longer required her

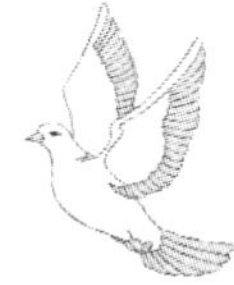

inhalers to breathe! I was amazed at the changes taking place in her health. Colds and illness were becoming less frequent.

A grand total of one asthma attack has occurred since she started with Chiropractic. Lauren is five years old now, having regular chiropractic adjustments, and is a healthy, happy little girl.

Thanks, Dr. Warner, for making all the difference to a family struggling with difficult choices for the health of their most precious gifts: their children.

ASHLEE'S STORY • *Ashlee's Mother*

Ashlee was born April 11, 1987, with Spastic Cerebral Palsy Triplegia. For some reason her umbilical cord was wrapped tightly around her little neck, not once, but three times. As a result, it caused severe trauma and many complications after birth.

I remember her birth as if it was just yesterday. The moment she was born I cried, mainly tears of joy, but there were some of sadness because I knew something was wrong. When the doctor showed me my little girl who was just minutes old, he did not let me hold her because she was so sick. In fact, I didn't get to hold my baby until Good Friday, when she was six days old. For the first five days I just got to touch her little hands and softly rub her little back. (Even to this day I still stand at my daughter's door and watch her sleep peacefully.)

So for the next little while, I knew something was wrong with Ashlee. I used to read books on the stages in a baby's life and look forward to her reaching those milestones. But, after months of the milestones passing her by, I knew for sure that something was wrong.

Ashlee was diagnosed with Cerebral Palsy on Friday, June 13, 1988, at 14 months. It was my parents who had to tell me because I was unable to go to her doctor's appointment. I think it probably was the hardest news that my parents had to tell me. That day I thought my world

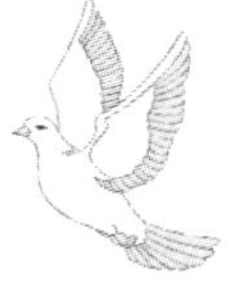

ended. I had no idea of what was going to happen to her, or even if she would live.

I only ever made one goal for Ashlee, to myself, and I said, "She'll walk by her second Christmas." This was after she was diagnosed. I never ever set any other goals for her in my mind, because when Christmas came and went she was just learning to crawl and I was so upset and depressed.

Ashlee started receiving physiotherapy at approximately eight months of age and she still gets weekly therapy from a physiotherapist and daily from us. As well, she also receives occupational therapy weekly.

At around 25 months of age, my dad and I took her to Toronto for an assessment. That is when I was told that it would be a miracle if she walked. Well, that miracle did happen at the age of three. On September 20, 1990, Ashlee took her first steps of unassisted walking. There was no stopping her now.

When Ashlee was five years old she had surgery on her left leg. This surgery (heal cord and hamstring lengthening) enabled Ashlee to walk with her little foot almost flat.

Before Ashlee began Chiropractic treatment with Dr. Tom, she was walking with a very noticeable gait. Her hips were not aligned at all. She hardly used her left hand. It was as if her left hand was just hanging there for decoration.

Now since receiving several months of treatment her walking/balance has improved a tremendous amount. Her hips are getting closer

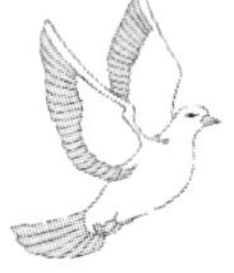

to being aligned and she uses her left arm/hand a lot more.

With all these changes happening with her, she is becoming more independent in her daily living activities. She can even take a shower. To quote Ashlee, "Baths are for little kids."

Because of her better balance/walking, I don't always have to be outside with her. This, in turn, means she can play with her friends without her mom looking over her shoulder all the time.

I truly believe Chiropractic care has given my daughter a new lease on a healthier, independent life. I would recommend Chiropractic care to all parents of physically challenged children. It gives children something that no other medical intervention has done or can do.

Thank you Doctor!

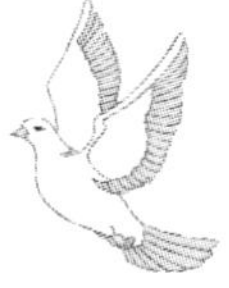

ASTHMA • *Donald J. Baune, D.C.*

Thank you for taking on such an adventure as your new book, Angie. I wish you luck and many blessings. I have had a miracle happen to me as a result of Chiropractic care that I would like to share with you.

I suffered from severe asthma as an infant. From the time I was born I had constant asthma attacks and was always in and out of the hospital and/or medical doctors' offices. I had to sleep on a slant with my head elevated. Someone had to watch me 24 hours around the clock because I would frequently stop breathing and they would then have to take me into the bathroom and turn on the hot water to let the steam open my blocked air passageways. I was constantly on medication and was getting worse, not better.

One day, when I was about one and a half years old, I was released from the hospital and my mother was told that they had done all that they could do for me. They suspected some type of wasting disease such as Hodgkin's disease and suggested some tests. They told her that it was just a matter of time now and that I probably had one to two months to live. She took me home and was very upset. That afternoon a neighbor came by and suggested to her again that she take me to Dr. Charles, a Chiropractor in Torrance. Since my mother was a nurse, she would never take her son to one of those quacks. This time, however, there was nothing to lose, so she took me to see him.

After examining and X-raying me, he determined that my atlas axis was jammed up against my skull. This seemed to make some sense to my mother, since during labor, I was starting to be born while she was still in the parking lot. The nurse put my mom on her side on a gurney, pushed me back in and sat on my mom's legs until they got her up to the delivery room.

Dr. Charles adjusted my atlas and sent me home. Within a few hours, I began coughing and spitting up tremendous amounts of phlegm. My mother said she could not believe there was that much inside such a small baby. I improved rapidly and within a week I was perfectly normal. The medical doctors could not believe it. When told it was due to Chiropractic care, they refused to give it any credit.

I continued to receive adjustments regularly the rest of my life and never even knew that I ever had a problem. I was very active in sports in high school and had no limitations whatsoever. When I was 17 years old, my mother told me the story. That's when I decided to become a Doctor of Chiropractic.

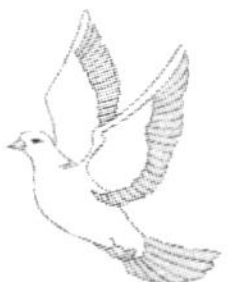

ASTHMA • *Leonard Cassara*

I was very sick with asthma and epilepsy which caused me to black out unexpectedly. I also suffered from headaches and severe allergic reactions to certain foods and substances. I was taking medication for my asthma three to four times every day before seeing the Chiropractor.

I had seen many other doctors, all to no avail. I felt very good about the initial consultation and examination by the Doctor of Chiropractic. It was very exciting when he told me he thought he could help me. I became hopeful.

Dr. Lawrence is very caring. He makes me feel very relaxed and at ease with his adjustments. At the present time I have had a tremendous change in the amount of times I need to take my asthma medication. From three to four times a day, I now take my medication only two to three times per month! No more headaches either. I feel good about myself and stronger too! Dr. Lawrence and his staff work with you. There is love in the air and it makes one feel good to be in the office!

I strongly advise anyone to seek Chiropractic care if they need or want to feel better in body, mind and spirit! Whatever condition you might have, try it! It will make a world of difference in your life and in your health.

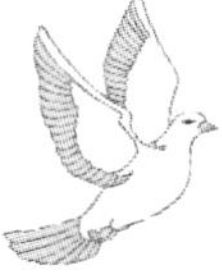

ASTHMA • *Rev. J. S. Hudley*

My three year old son Byron had been suffering with asthma for many months. We had taken him to several doctors. They would only give him shots or medicine that didn't help. The shots would last about eight hours and then he would wheeze and cough worse than before. We were taking him to the doctor two and three times a week.

Sometimes he would wheeze and cough so hard, he would hardly sleep at night. Some attacks would last for two or three weeks. Then a friend told me about Chiropractic. I took Byron to the chiropractor. He took an X-ray of his spine and explained to me about the misalignments that were causing his asthma.

After his first three adjustments we could see amazing results, and Byron seemed like a new child. Now, after one year of Chiropractic adjustments, Byron has had only one bad asthma attack. I can truly say, "Thank God for Chiropractic."

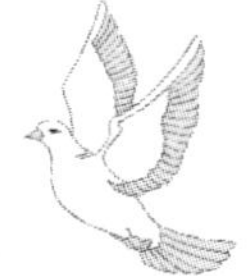

ASTHMA • *Linda and Mark*

Dear Doctor,

When we brought Michael to you for the first time at about 11 months old, he was already diagnosed as having asthma and on three different medications. His face was always red because he never stopped wheezing. We used to take him to the hospital quite often to be given shots and put on a machine to breathe better. After just a few Chiropractic adjustments he was able to breathe and we slowly weaned him off all his medications. He was then able to sleep through the night—which he had never done before—and was much more comfortable.

Now, at the age of three, he no longer has any breathing problems. We take him once a month for an adjustment. His body speaks to him to tell him when he needs another adjustment.

Thank you for all your help!

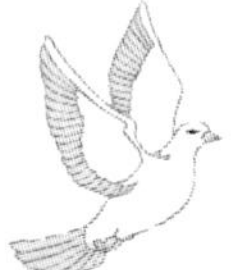

ASTHMA • *Mrs. Martha E. McCoy*

Ever since my son was born, he has been bothered with terrible asthma attacks. His attacks were so severe that he would have to be rushed to the hospital and given oxygen. His attacks seemed to be in regular intervals, but would he get so much worse during the cold weather. I tried all kinds of medicine and vaporizers with no results whatsoever. It would just tear my heart to pieces to hear my boy wheezing and gasping for breath.

Upon the advice of my parents, I took my son to the chiropractor. His examination revealed the cause of his trouble. He said my son could be helped. In just a few weeks time, his asthma seemed to be better. It has now been eight months since the chiropractor first adjusted him. He has had only one slight attack in this time.

I am thankful to Chiropractic for giving me a healthy son. I sure would advise people who are sick to try Chiropractic. It works!

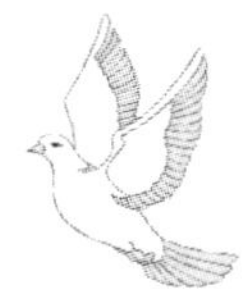

ATTENTION DEFICIT DISORDER

• *Elana Brown, D.C.*

Sheldon was born in 1936 to Polish immigrant parents, the youngest of five children. His parents were told this child is a "vegetable." He would not live very long but if he did, he would not amount to much because his capabilities are limited.

When he was small, he was beautiful. At four years of age, he had soft, blonde, curly hair and big blue eyes. He was deaf and had no speech. He was unable to learn. He wouldn't sit still and would run around the house screaming while holding his head between his hands. In fact, if you wanted him to move you had to push him in the direction he was supposed to go.

My father was already a friend of the family. His friend was the older brother of Sheldon. My father had not yet married my mother, Sheldon's sister. My father had been brought out of paralysis by Chiropractic and he told the family that they should take this boy to a chiropractor. He didn't know what kind of response the child would have, but knew that Chiropractic could only help.

The family finally agreed. They took him to a local man named Louis Martell. This chiropractor took an X-ray of Sheldon's spine and found that the first bone in the neck was rotated over 45 degrees. The chiropractor adjusted him. The neck released beautifully. From that adjustment, the boy was able to sit

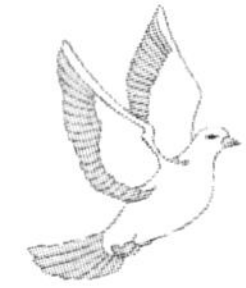

still. He did not run around the house screaming or holding his head between his hands. In fact, he was now ready to learn language. His two sisters went to the New York Society of the Deaf to learn sign language in order to teach him.

Today he is 60 years of age. He has outlasted his parents and siblings. He is an artist who has painted about 100 paintings. The sad part is that he lost 16 years of developmental skills that are so crucial to a developing child. But he is a sweetheart, a very mild mannered and kind person.

Chiropractic is very much a part of his life. He has received regular adjustments more often if he felt a cold or flu symptoms. He hasn't taken aspirins or antibiotics since he was 16 years old.

On one occasion he came in saying, "My social worker was out sick today. Doesn't she know about Chiropractic?" Even with his limited mental ability, he understands that Chiropractic is important to keep him healthy. Shouldn't we all?

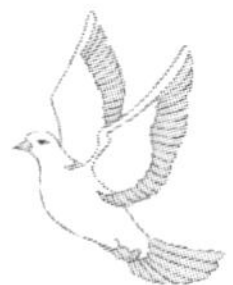

ATTENTION DEFICIT DISORDER

• *Stephen R. Goldman, D.C.*

A two-year-old child had a medical diagnosis of "developmental community disorder." He was non-responsive to any external stimuli, even to receiving an injection. His abnormal symptoms started at birth.

On examination, he kept repeating hand motions and strange grunts and did not respond to sound or touch. Chiropractic analysis showed an axis subluxation and I was unable to test for spinal stress areas.

On the third visit when I walked into the room, he began to cry. This was the first time that he responded to anything happening around him. By the sixth adjustment, he started to follow certain commands and stopped making repeated hand motions. He started to talk after the twelfth office visit. At present, he has an extensive vocabulary and is slightly hyperactive.

He is probably making up for lost time.

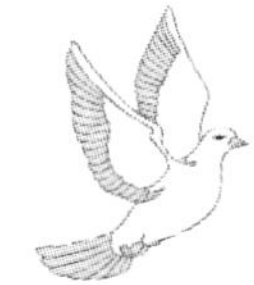

AUTISM • *Kevin and Lynne Grobsky*

Our son Thomas was born on September 22, 1989. Although his rate of development was slow, he was still within the normal parameters. He smiled and made the usual baby noises and was a happy, healthy child. We became concerned when his verbal skills had not yet emerged by the age of two. By that time he had stopped making noises. Our pediatrician suggested that Tom suffered from global developmental delays. Shortly after this diagnosis, we moved to Connecticut and subsequently enrolled Tom in an early intervention program at the age of three. Finally after a short period, Tom was diagnosed with autism.

Prior to the age of three, Tommy had not shown any autistic symptoms of which we were aware. However, from the age of three on his symptoms got markedly worse in spite of early intervention. These symptoms included lack of vocalization, aggression, sleep disturbances, mild self abuse, frequent temper tantrums and general lack of interest in toys. Under the guidance of a wonderful special education teacher, Tommy showed improvement in his social skills, verbal skills and social development. However, his aggression and temper tantrums continued to worsen.

His aggressiveness increased to such an extent that we decided to enlist the help of a behavioral psychologist. After a time, his behavior improved and his autism became more marked.

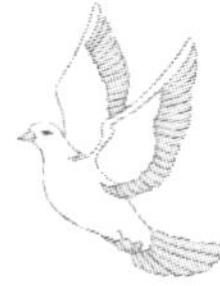

We read as many books as we could on autism in order to help our son as much as possible. In all the information we reviewed, no one told us that Chiropractic could be a tool in the treatment of autism. When we heard from a friend of successes in treating children with special needs, we decided to give it a try. The fact that Chiropractic is non-invasive and drug - free made it especially attractive.

We made an appointment in November 1996. The day after his first adjustment was the best day that Tommy had ever had. He played with toys all day and his interactive speech increased dramatically. He actually played with his sister! The change in him has been truly remarkable. Although he still has his ups and his downs, his downs are so much less severe.

The overall improvement of his cognitive and social development has been dramatic. He is now learning to read! His average grades in his general class have gone from 70% to 86% in six months. His classmates interact with him to a much greater extent. He also eats a wider variety of foods and his sleep disturbances are markedly reduced.

There is no doubt in our minds that Chiropractic has been instrumental in reducing Tommy's autistic symptoms!

Thank you Dr. DiRubba!

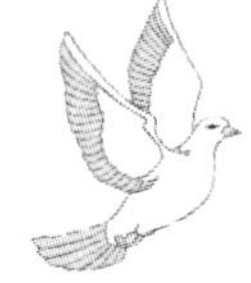

BETTER THAN BACK SURGERY

• *Ira L. Ford Jr.*

One day, while bending over to pick up a tire, I felt something snap in my back. A pain hit me so bad I could hardly get up. The pain was so bad I had to be helped into my car and driven home. That night I had to take pain pills, but could not rest and I felt worse. On Sunday I felt so bad that my wife called a bone specialist. He had me admitted to the hospital that day and put me in traction with 50 pounds of weight. While in the hospital I was given shots of Demerol to keep me comfortable and a physiotherapist treated me every day.

After one week of this I was no better, in fact, I was worse. The specialist finally told me that if I was not better the next day, he would operate on me. That day I got permission to leave the hospital on personal business. My wife put me in a wheel chair and took me to see a chiropractor. I had heard about Chiropractic and thought I would try it before letting anyone cut into my spine. With my wife's help, I got to the chiropractor's office.

The doctor examined my spine, found the cause of my trouble and corrected it. He then told me to get up and walk. I was afraid to, but I tried it and to my amazement the pain was gone. I then returned to the hospital and got back in bed. After a while the specialist came and checked me. He was amazed at how well I was doing. He told me I could go home.

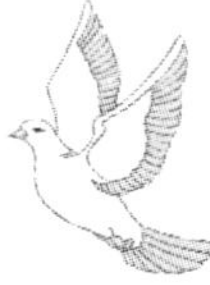

Just think, if I hadn't tried Chiropractic I may have been disabled for life. I am very thankful for what the chiropractor has done for me.

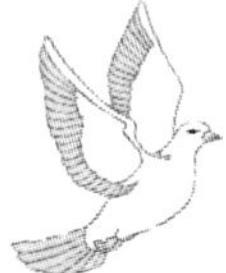

BED-WETTING • *Marie and Adam*

My son, Adam, is a nine-year-old, energetic, bright 'A' student, aspiring artist and a boy who loves the outdoors. Adam, however, has a problem. He wets his bed. Adam has had this problem for a while and had to endure the teasing from his five brothers and sisters, two of whom are younger than he is and are not bedwetters.

Staying overnight at friends, going camping or even visiting relatives in Canada was embarrassing for Adam because he always had to take along his "diapers." We became so concerned about this problem that I asked a few medical doctors for their advice. Their answer was that Adam would probably out-grow the problem. We were also told to "cut down on his fluid intake just before bed time." We tried that; it didn't work. We even went to the extreme of embarrassing him even more by telling him we would tell his teachers and all his friends at school. Poor Adam! He really tried to control his bladder, but he still wet his bed at night.

It wasn't until a good friend recommended County Line Chiropractic Center to me for some problems I was having that I decided to see if Chiropractic adjustments would help Adam also. The adjustments were helping me, but would they really help Adam control his bladder at night? I had doubts which immediately flew out the window the morning after Adam had his first adjustment with Dr. Bob. I went

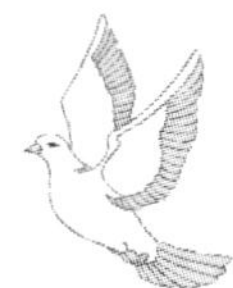

into his room as usual to wake him up for school and noticed he was wearing the same pajamas he had put on for bed the night before. We were all so happy, we hugged him and cheered him on. I was so happy that I cried and wondered if this could be the end of Adam's bed-wetting problem.

Well, it has been over one month that Adam has been seeing Dr. Bob and his wonderful staff. I am very proud to say that Adam has not wet his bed once since his adjustments started. I thank God for allowing me to meet Dr. Bob and his staff, who with their bright smiles and warm welcome always make us feel good about ourselves.

We thank you Dr. Bob!

BED-WETTING • *Jonathon's Mother*

My five-year-old son Jon had a constant problem with bladder control. He wet his pants both day and night. Jon has always been a very active, healthy boy.

We tried reward charts, thinking that the positive encouragement would help him remember to use the toilet. He was raised on natural, "whole" foods and vitamins, and was breast fed. When junk food did sift into his diet, we made a rule – NO sugars. That also made little difference. We always tried to attack the problem, but not Jon. The problem was Jon's bladder not the person Jon. I believe this is why Jon's self esteem has been high although he has been in many embarrassing situations.

We decided to try Chiropractic care after I had talked to a number of different chiropractors. They all agreed that Chiropractic care helped with bed-wetting.

After talking with Dr. Henry, and as a result of his encouragement, we decided to try Chiropractic care. Jon's X-rays showed that the nerves that relate to the bladder were being compressed by a vertebrae that was out of line. This caused the normal signals from the bladder to the brain to be interrupted, resulting in Jon being unaware of the need to urinate.

Jon's problem never caused much of an interruption in his hobbies of swimming, biking, and general play. Having constant wet pants caused him a lot of embarrassment at school.

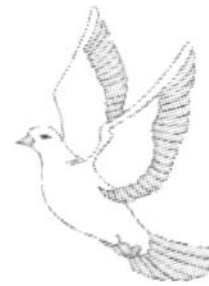

After six months of treatment, John stays dry during the day. Some nights are still a problem, but they are fewer than the dry nights. Now Jon wakes up with a smile in a dry bed and says, "I didn't wet!"

I would encourage all parents who are concerned about their child's bed-wetting problem to try the Chiropractic approach. I know that Jon has a special respect for his Chiropractic Doctor and thinks the world of him.

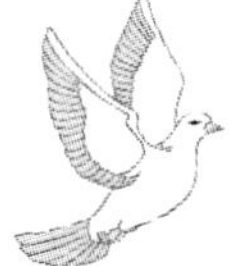

BLINDNESS • *G. Hartman, D.C.*

The Amazing Story of George James

When George James consulted our Chiropractic office because of severe headaches and neck pains, he received much more than he expected. George had been blind in his right eye for 17 years and had given up hope that anything could be done to restore his vision. In fact, he lived with his disability for so long that he did not even mention it. Yet, the evening after his first Chiropractic adjustment his eyesight miraculously began returning. Here is George's story:

At age 16, George woke up one morning to discover that he had lost the vision in his right eye. Shocked and dismayed at this sudden loss, his mother immediately made arrangements for him to be examined at Will's Eye Hospital in Philadelphia. After extensive testing, the doctors announced that they could not find the reason for his loss of sight.

For an entire year George continued to return for follow-up exams hoping the doctors would find the source of his problem. Later he consulted a neurosurgeon who suggested that he might be suffering from multiple sclerosis which could account for his visual disturbance.

Finally George was referred to another renowned eye specialist in Philadelphia. Again, exhaustive testing and examination procedures were undertaken. The doctor had to honestly

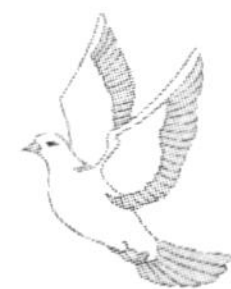

and regretfully inform George that there was no known medical reason for his loss of vision.

Discouraged, George feared a life of disability and gradual deterioration from his suspected multiple sclerosis. For some twelve years longer he lived with his problem, always expecting the worst.

Then he woke up one morning with a severe headache and terrible neck pain. "Aspirins wouldn't even begin to touch it," he said. A very close friend suggested that he see a chiropractor. She felt sure that he could help George with his headaches and neck pains.

George was skeptical, never having considered this type of treatment before. The pain continued and George finally consented to give this new doctor a try. After all, what did he have to lose? Things couldn't get much worse! George called for his first appointment.

After a careful case history and examination, his spine was X-rayed to determine the possibility of spinal nerve pressure. The films confirmed the presence of serious vertebral subluxations (pinched nerves) that were apparently causing his headaches and neck pains.

After his first corrective spinal adjustment, George began to experience some relief. The next evening was when the "Miracle" occurred. George was watching television when his right eye "flashed with sight for about a half hour." It then faded away once again. Puzzled and frightened, George didn't tell anyone at first. The next day his vision returned again and stayed, getting clearer and stronger.

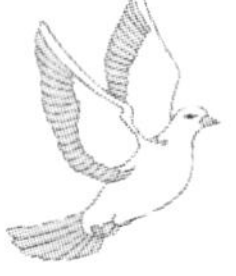

George visited his chiropractor two days later and not only reported the improvement in his head and neck pain but also the return of vision in his right eye. "The doctor was almost speechless," George said. "He covered my left eye and gave me a brochure to read which I did without difficulty. He gave me another one at random and I was able to read that one as well."

George had a comprehensive eye examination several weeks later which showed the visual acuity in his right eye to be 20/30, almost normal. His vision has continued to improve since then, his most recent reading in his formerly "blind" eye being 20/22.

Like George, the first chiropractic patient, Harvey Lillard, had a serious functional impairment corrected by Chiropractic. He had been deaf for 17 years and had his hearing restored by the first Chiropractic adjustment. Since then over 55 million people have benefited from Chiropractic care, not only to correct health problems, but also to maintain the best possible health and well-being.

This does not mean to imply that all visual disturbances can benefit from Chiropractic care. However, George's experience underscores the fact that many functional and metabolic disturbances are a direct result of "pinched nerves" in the spinal column. Truly it is proper to say: "Everything possible has not been done unless Chiropractic has been included."

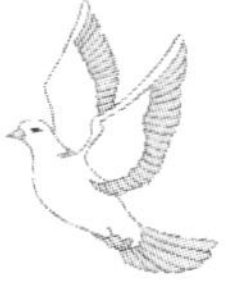

BLINDNESS • *R.N., D.C.*

I am a second generation chiropractor. I recently treated one of my father's patients who told me about his miracle.

In 1950 or there abouts, a young man, who was 14 years old at the time, had a serious head injury which rendered him blind.

After several months of medical treatment he was brought to my dad for Chiropractic treatment. After two Chiropractic upper cervical adjustments, his sight returned. He has been going to my dad ever since. Miracles happen every day.

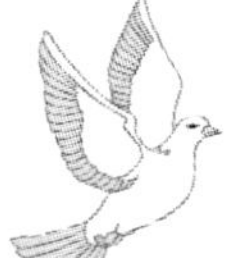

BLURRED VISION • *Sheri F.*

One morning in November 1994 my daughter Nina awoke with the vision in both of her eyes blurred from the bridge of her nose down. Instead of this condition abating, it worsened as the day wore on. We saw her pediatrician first. He had never seen or heard of such a sudden onset of blurred vision without the display of other symptoms. He referred us to an ophthalmologist.

That afternoon the blurred vision finally went away, although Nina was left with an inability to focus. When she made the effort to focus, words were shaky and her eyes were achy from muscle strain.

The ophthalmologist examined Nina extensively and he also said he had not heard or read anything in the literature that could explain what was happening. Her optic nerve and the rest of the physiology around the eye appeared healthy and normal. Her vision was 20/25 despite her inability to focus. In other words, I was being left to my own devises to figure out how to "fix" the problem as well as discovering what the problem was in the first place.

Meanwhile, the implications for our daughter's future flooded our brains. My eight-year-old was beginning to worry, as we had been to well-respected and competent doctors and an eye specialist and had been told "the cupboard is bare," so to speak. We had no answers.

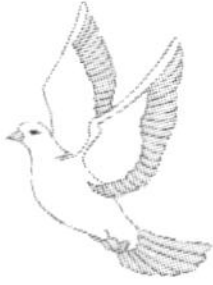

I happened to have an appointment that evening with Dr. Ornelas, my chiropractor, directly after the appointment with the ophthalmologist. I jokingly said to my daughter, "Wouldn't it be funny if Dr. Ornelas adjusted you and everything went back to normal?" I had my usual adjustment and I then asked Dr. Ornelas to take a look at Nina. I figured we had exhausted the initial medical aspects so it couldn't hurt to try this, too.

Dr. Ornelas discovered the right side of Nina's neck was sorely out of alignment. Upon questioning Nina, she realized the area around the right eye tended to be the most tender by the end of each day. Dr. Ornelas made only one neck adjustment and iced the area for about five minutes.

Within 15 minutes we were walking into our house and suddenly I heard Nina scream loudly. She discovered that she could see clearly and normally again. We had left a cracker box on the kitchen counter that morning and she was reading the ingredients label. She was so excited that she was running around our house reading everything.

We had just gone through five days of staying up late at night completing homework and worrying about what the future was to hold for a child with special sight needs and possibly other physical problems (brain tumors?). When I realized Nina's vision had returned to normal, I can't express the relief I felt.

When trying to think of possible causes for

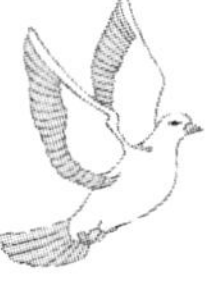

Nina's condition, we could implicate normal rough play at school or a fall from her loft bed two weeks earlier.

I shudder to think of the time, energy, expense and possible surgery that we could have gone through in trying to find a cause and a cure. The medical community that we dealt with did a wonderful job for us. We felt we were being cared for by very dedicated people. However, they never mentioned Chiropractic as an option to explore. I feel very strongly that there is indeed a place for Chiropractic care in a well-rounded health maintenance program. I'm glad that Chiropractic was an option we exercised early in this case as it saved us much discomfort and inconvenience, as well as possible permanent damage for our child.

Thanks Dr. Ornelas !!!!!

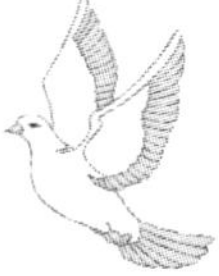

BLURRED VISION

• *Stephen R. Goldman, D.C.*

A 77-year-old patient's main complaint was blurred vision and double vision that occurred on and off throughout the day. An examination by a neuro-ophthalmic specialist resulted in a diagnosis of ocular myothenia. The patient refused medical therapy for this condition.

Chiropractic analysis showed an axis subluxation. After four adjustments, the patient experienced a reduction in symptoms. She no longer had any symptoms by the ninth visit. She is presently under maintenance care and has not had a recurrence of her problem.

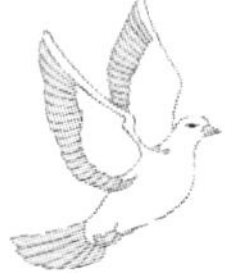

CANCER • *Jean Wetterlin, D.C.*

My name is Jean Brown Wetterlin, D. C. The D. C. stands for "Doctor of Chiropractic." It's because of the basic beliefs that Chiropractic is founded on that I am alive today. I was diagnosed, during surgery for what my medical doctor thought would be a routine removal of benign muscle tumors of the uterus, with polysystic adeno carcinoma, stage 3-C. What this means is that I have a very advanced case of ovarian cancer. This happened on October 23, 1992.

During this surgery, removal of my ovaries omentum (the outer fat layer that protects your pelvis between your hips), uterus, tubes and residual tumor that they could get to, took place. I was told that my right ovary was the size of a volleyball and that my left ovary was about grapefruit size and had grown into the pelvic wall. The only symptom I had observed was an odd feeling (no pain) in the lower left quadrant of my pelvis. This was probably due to the left ovary beginning to pull away from the wall of the pelvis as that tumor grew and gained weight. My surgeon did take out as much tumor as she could; however, there was still tumor left in me. The places mentioned in the surgical report were as follows: on top of the bowel, in the base of the pelvis, implants of three to five centimeters under my diaphragm and on top of the dome of the liver. The fluids of the pelvis tested positive as well.

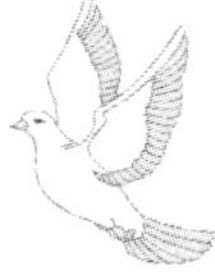

After surgery, I was sent to an ob-gyn oncologist at the University of Minnesota who reviewed my case, pathology reports and did a physical examination. I was then told that I had one year to live; six months without pain. He recommended that I get started with chemotherapy right away to gain additional "months." I told him that I was a Chiropractor, believed in the body's ability to heal itself, and was considering alternative recommendations. The oncologist blatantly told me that if I did not follow his advice I would be back within six months in severe pain, begging him for what he had to offer. Needless to say, over the next two weeks I struggled with what decision I should make. What I decided was based on the fact that I would not let fear dictate my choice, but rather I would make my decision on what I know to be true.

Chiropractic espouses that the body has within it an intelligence to care for itself. It is a natural occurrence and is able to function, without help, as long as there is no interference. I looked at my life and started to unload the garbage and baggage I was carrying—mentally, emotionally and physically. I decided to go to Jaurez, Mexico to a facility called the International Medical Center where I was evaluated and examined and started on a regimen of care for one month. This routine included procedures that are considered non-invasive and enhancing to the body: ozone therapy, laitril (vitamin B17, which is illegal in the U.S.), nutritional considerations and organic

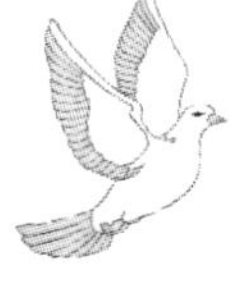

sources, shark cartilage both orally and rectally, coffee enemas, reike machine, aloe vera, thalamine and fetal animal cell shots to stimulate the immune system to kick in. As well, there were Chiropractic adjustments, colonic therapy, massive dosages of vitamins, and massage and hydrotherapy for relaxation. Each patient at the Center was treated individually.

While there I also saw another doctor outside the Center who was using a product that a nuclear physicist invented. The physicist had been employed by the U.S. government and was retired. He developed intestinal cancer with the same cell-type that I had (adenocarcinoma). Everything that I did had the basic premise of helping my body to help itself and worked with enhancing my body's own abilities to heal.

As of last December, all blood tests showed no cancer growth, and even the most intricate imaging done by MRI and CT scans show no cancer. These past three and one-half years have been relatively pain free. I've been able to continue my work as a Chiropractor and live my life to the fullest. I am tracked by a pelvic oncologist in St. Paul who shakes his head at me and says that in twenty years of practice he has never seen another case such as mine. I am writing a book that will probably be named IT'S THE BIG "C" ... AND IT DOESN'T STAND FOR CANCER, which hopefully will be finished before my five-year survival date!

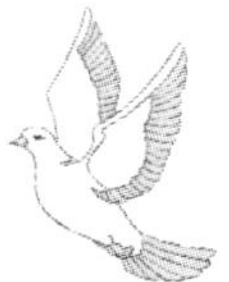

CEREBRAL PALSY • *Alla Gershburg*

My son Mitchell has cerebral palsy and for the past six months has had seizures which last all day. Prior to Chiropractic treatment, Mitchell had no previous treatment or results. We never gave him medication as we believe it is harmful to the brain.

Upon reading an article about Chiropractic helping a person with epilepsy, we decided to see a chiropractor. We had our doubts that Chiropractic would work; however, our first impression of Dr. Sirlin and his office was wonderful!

Dr. Sirlin recommended to continue the adjustments on a weekly basis and the seizures stopped IMMEDIATELY!!

Presently, all four of us in our family are chiropractic patients for backaches, arthritis and prevention of any illness. As a matter of fact, our daughter had chronic ear infections and her adjustments have helped her almost instantly.

I would recommend to anyone sick or suffering in pain to try Chiropractic and see whether it works for them. I have told everyone I know that Chiropractic is the alternative care for many, many conditions and a great preventive measure.

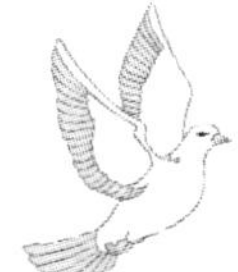

CHRON'S DISEASE • *E.K., D.C.*

A 31-year-old patient had a diagnosis of Chron's disease, with which he had struggled for 15 years. A portion of his intestine had been removed, and he was taking an antibiotic and prednisone. From the time his symptoms began, he never experienced a normal bowel movement and was constantly suffering from abdominal cramps. He also complained of extreme weakness and an inability to put on weight.

Chiropractic analysis showed a subluxation of the axis. His spine stabilized on the fifth visit. By the sixth visit, he started feeling better and his medication was reduced. He started to have normal bowel movements by the thirteenth visit, and all medication was stopped. I examine this patient every three weeks. He has no abnormal gastrointestinal symptoms, and his weight and strength have greatly improved.

Along with adjustments, it was also necessary to alter his diet by removing certain foods that are known irritants to patients with this condition.

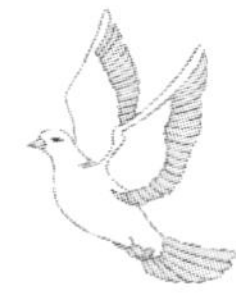

CHRONIC DISEASES • *Judy Blondin*

My Chiropractic Story – 1995

Today I enjoy a full life. I enjoy the outdoors through wilderness canoeing (including portaging) and cross country skiing. It was not always that way. Before I found Chiropractic care my life was pain and sickness.

In 1978 my life was filled with pain: severe headaches, upper- and low-back pain, severe knee pain, chronic bronchitis.

I had headaches for ten years, and they were getting worse each year. I consulted a medical doctor and was given many different kinds of prescription pain pills. None of these helped, including a brain scan, which was negative.

I had upper thoracic pain so severe (especially when pregnant) that a heating pad went with me wherever I went.

My low back pain of ten-year duration was becoming worse each year and gradually moving into my left leg and hip. I could not get out of bed in the morning for pain. Each morning my husband would rub my lower back so I could move without feeling like I was breaking in half.

Knee pain was so severe I could not walk down stairs. Usually I slid down on my behind. I could not stand for any length of time to prepare dinner or do any outside sports with my family. A rheumatoid and arthritic specialist told me I had muscular rheumatism in my knees and I would have to learn to live with this pain. There was nothing wrong with me. My medical doctor

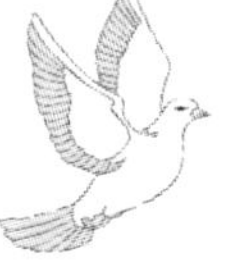

injected cortisone into my knees without helping. I also tried self-hypnotism without results.

With having chronic bronchitis, I was constantly on medication. The regular dosage needed to be doubled to effect a cure. A side effect from so much medication was that I caught every virus. I had bronchitis every month. I smoked two packs of cigarettes a day; I quit on December 5, 1979. I still got bronchitis. This was supposedly triggered by allergies. At this time in my life allergy injections were taken monthly for three years.

My lucky day came in 1979 when I began to work for a chiropractor. He began regular treatments. Headaches and back problems eased up.

In 1980 I started to work for Dr. Hollingsworth, D.C., who besides Chiropractic training, had taken additional courses in Applied Kinesiology and Podiatry. He was able to help me even more! My headaches disappeared, with a slight attack now and then. Knee pain was gone in two weeks. I stopped allergy injections in late 1980. Now when I feel a spasm or heavy feeling in my chest, I get a chiropractic adjustment warding off a bronchial attack.

With my past experience in Chiropractic care, I am totally committed to the natural way to good health with Chiropractic care as my first choice. I recommend regular Chiropractic care to maintain a healthy life.

I firmly believe I am here today because of Chiropractic care!

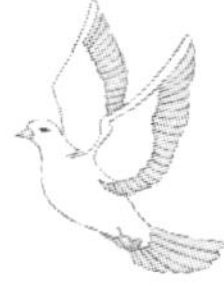

CHRONIC INFECTION • *S.W., D.C.*

A 22-month-old child was diagnosed as having chronic infection and febrile seizures. This condition started when he fell out of a chair and hit his head on the floor. He had been given antibiotics and phenobarbital since six months of age. As a result of the medication, he did not eat well and lacked the strength to play with other children.

Chiropractic analysis showed a subluxation of the atlas. After the third adjustment, his medication was gradually reduced. By the fifth adjustment, his blood count was normal and there was no indication of infection. This was the first negative blood test in a year. Within four months, all medication was stopped and he resumed normal activities for a boy of his age.

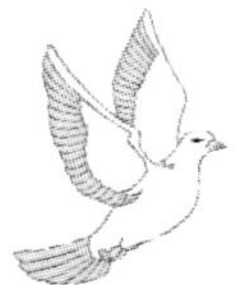

CHRONIC PAIN • *Cheryl Moger*

I'm a school bus driver and have driven a standard school bus for the past four years. Unbeknown to me I was developing a hip disorder. The constant repetitive use of my left leg on the clutch was causing daily pain in my hip which spread up into my lower back.

This pain, which I thought was due to the normal aging process, started slowly and was very minimal and gradually escalated to a very sharp stabbing pain. I was finding it very difficult to even walk around the block. The pain was unbearable!

This was very disturbing to me as summer was almost here and our family likes to go places and do things. Since I did not want to cancel any outings because of me, I decided I was going to do something about this pain and not let this condition get the best of me.

I've been receiving Chiropractic adjustments for three months now and I'm very pleased to say that we recently walked around Ontario Place for hours, and I did it pain free. Yahoo! Thank you very much!

Without Chiropractic care, I wonder what condition I'd be in ten years from now. I strongly believe that Chiropractic care enhances the quality of life.

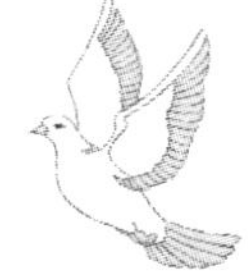

CHRONIC PAIN • *Kim Lung*

After seeing Noel's presentation at Home Depot, I started to think about the chronic pain I put up with in my knee. I was considering having surgery again to correct the way the joint was moving. I decided to give Chiropractic a try. Anything was better than surgery and the rehabilitation that inevitably follows.

Surprisingly, my knee improved almost right away, but even more surprising was that my headaches were also getting less frequent and less intense. Another benefit was that I began to get less monthly cramps and my menstrual cycle began to balance out. Overall I've had more energy and less pain after overdoing things at work. I don't panic anymore if my migraine medication isn't in my purse. You can't imagine how liberating that is! I'm spending less money on pain killers and anti-inflammatories now.

I had seen a few other chiropractors in the past, but only for a back injury sustained at work. I think the difference with this particular office is the dynamic atmosphere that permeates their open, educational approach to subluxation elimination. Noel's willingness to explain and show how everything works made me feel a part of the healing process rather than just a recipient of a treatment. Everyone in the office feels like family, and that certainly makes a critical difference for me. I sleep, work and play better than I ever thought I could without surgery.

I'm glad I took the Chiropractic plunge!

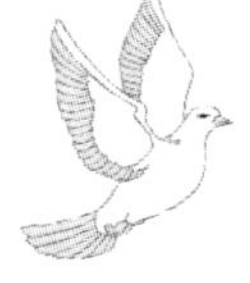

CHRONIC PAIN • *Juliette Guilbert*

I first went to see my chiropractor because of severe muscular pain in my right shoulder, which I had been experiencing for a year. Looking back on that year, I am amazed at how readily I submitted to the idea that constant pain was normal. I remember thinking that it must be a result of getting older (I'm 29 now), and that I would just have to get used to it since it could only get worse as I approached middle age. This was a gloomy attitude for an otherwise healthy woman, but there was no other explanation to my problem. I exercised, ate sensibly, tried to maintain good health, and did everything I knew to stay healthy.

During the initial examination, it became abundantly clear to me that a chiropractor's approach was different from any version of medicine I had previously experienced.

I was impressed that even before any X-rays were taken, he put his hand on exactly the place that felt like the center of my upper back pain. He also identified two spots—one in my midback and one in my lower back—that had bothered me to a greater or lesser degree for years. However, he offered me no explanations or theories about the pain, nor did he make any inflated claims as to what he could do for me.

This contrasted sharply with the approach of most doctors that I had been to see who asked me a million questions, theorized about the causes of the problems or symptoms, and

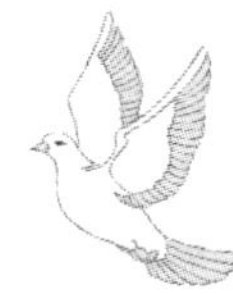

seemed abundantly confident that they could give my problems a name. There was, however, no relief from them, even after drugs and therapy.

After my first adjustment, the pain in my back completely disappeared for the first time in over a year. For the next two days as my body detoxed, I felt as though I had the flu. Only then did I fully realize how awful the previous year had been and that it hadn't been normal at all. After the first adjustment the pain returned in a cyclically diminishing way, but was never as severe again. Now after three months, the pain is almost completely gone. I still get the occasional twinge if I have to drive a lot but that is all. I never imagined that this pain could be related to my spine.

I have suffered from chronic and sometimes debilitating pain in my right foot for about three years. The orthopedic specialists at Yale-New Haven Hospital had diagnosed this pain as the result of an "assory-novicular bone." The remedy being the insertion of a $150 cork. If the cork did not work, they said that they would have to shave the bone down to an acceptable size and shape.

After two Chiropractic adjustments, I began to make connections that had never occurred to me before. All of my pain was down the right side of my body—right foot, right hip, right shoulder—and it amazes me that no one else saw this fact as noteworthy. Then it began to dawn on me that the entire right side of my body hurt.

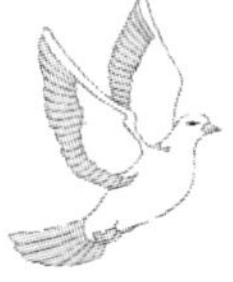

I took the orthopedic insert out of my shoe and was delighted to find that my novicular pain diminished after only a few adjustments. It rarely bothers me now. I feel confident that this condition, like my back pain, will continue to improve as my body adjusts and gets stronger. I have also lost weight and feel more energetic and positive.

I no longer feel as though I have one foot in the grave. Hurrah for Chiropractic!

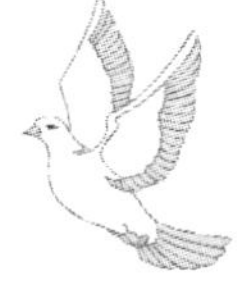

COSTOCHONDRITIS

• *Michael Budincick, D.C.*

Many of us in the Chiropractic field take for granted that most of our patients get well or better on a regular basis for the various types of neuromusculoskeletal conditions that we treat. Most of the symptoms that we see involve the lower back and neck pain.

Since this seems to be the most common complaint of the patients that visit us, many of us lose sight of the major conditions that are suffered by humanity.

One such case entered my office on the Saturday before Christmas 1993. The day after Thanksgiving the younger brother of Cody, my patient, jumped up to hug his brother. He hugged him from behind, striking him sharply in the back of the head and moving his head forward. Cody immediately reported neck pain to his mother, but continued to play with continued stiffness through the day. For several days he continued to complain of intermittent pain and the inability to move his neck, particularly when he was sitting, reading or watching television.

Upon his return to California, Cody was taken to Pasadena where X-rays were taken of his neck. The doctor reported that he saw nothing wrong, but sent the X-rays out for a reading anyway. He gave Cody a soft collar and told him to use heat packs. The X-ray came back negative, but when Cody took the neck brace off he reported that he felt "loose," and had difficulty

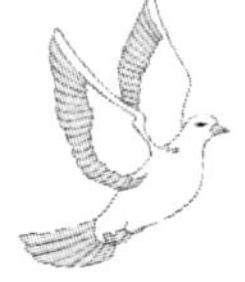

holding his neck upright. During the next five days, he continued to have episodes of moderate to severe pain in his neck.

Several days later at a day care center, Cody collapsed on a couch with the apparent symptoms of the flu or a systemic problem. On December 11 he complained of his whole body aching, and by evening was only able to walk when assisted. After having severe chest pain he was rushed to Antelope Valley Hospital Emergency. He was X-rayed for the chest pain, given blood tests and was diagnosed as having "Costochondritis." When the doctors were asked why Cody couldn't walk, they said that they did not know.

Two days later the parents rushed Cody to the hospital. When the nurse discovered that he had lost the feeling in the bottoms of his feet and several of his fingers, it was decided that he should be admitted into hospital. For the next five days he was examined by neurologists and internists, had a spinal tap, a cervical and head MRI, as well as several other X-rays. By this time he could hardly hold his head up and was unable to lift his arms to feed himself.

On Cody's parents carried his limp body into my office along with his X-rays. They were distraught and seeing a Doctor of Chiropractor was their last resort. I examined his body and found his reflexes to be normal with no apparent atrophy. The boy was unable to move any muscle or speak above a whisper.

Motion palpation revealed an extremely

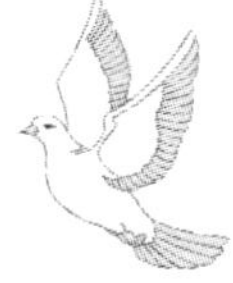

tender and locked right occiptal condyle area. Review of the X-rays showed extreme lateralisation of the atlas with lateral tilt, indicative of atlantaloccipital subluxation. With consent of his parents, I adjusted the right condyle.

Within minutes the boy was able to move his feet and hands. His headache completely disappeared. That night he was put in a hot tub at his parent's house and began to move and steadily improve.

Two days later, when his parents took him in for his next adjustment, he was able to sit up and he had written a Christmas card thanking me and expressing his appreciation for his improvement. His parents continued the in-water exercises for another two days. When he came into the office again, he had feeling in the bottom of his feet and hands and could walk with some assistance.

In a week he could walk by himself and he was improving daily. Just eleven days after his first adjustment, Cody was trying on his new rollerblades and was seen by his parents climbing a tree in his back yard.

The doctors at the hospital had no medical explanation and indicated that the problem was probably in the boy's head. His parents wrote that in the spring he began to play ball in the "Little League."

Many Chiropractors would ask the question whether they would treat him or refer him. We all know the innate power of Chiropractic when miracles are performed.

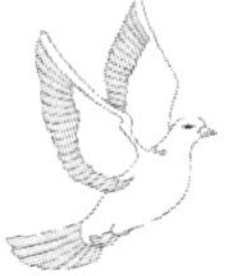

DANNY'S STORY • *The Cooper Family*

May 7, 1992

We were referred to a chiropractor for my son Danny who had a very bad year with asthma. Right before we started going, Danny had strep throat and a very bad wheeze. He was put on antibiotics, a cortisone inhaler twice a day, a Proventil inhaler every 4-6 hours and liquid Proventil between uses of the inhaler. He was put on a machine to open his passageways three times before he finally started breathing a little better, but he was still wheezing.

His pediatrician also wanted to put him on cortisone pills for a few days, but I refused because I didn't want him on any more medicine. We were back and forth to the doctor constantly to treat his wheeze. They always said that he was better, but he still had a slight wheeze. He has never really breathed right since he was two years old when his asthma started. He missed many days of school and many classes of Tae Kwon Do because he just couldn't breathe.

Luckily for us my husband started talking to Roy at the Tae Kwon Do class about Danny's asthma. Roy told us about a chiropractor who helped his son get rid of his asthma and his strep throats. We thought we should go too.

By the third adjustment, Danny told the Doctor of Chiropractic that he could breathe! He said, "My asthma is gone!"

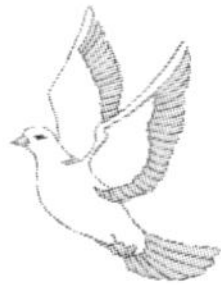

After going for a month, we went to my father's house for Passover. He has a long-haired dog that sometimes bothers Danny's breathing. Danny started wheezing and the chiropractor told us to come right over to his house at 10:00 p.m.

He adjusted him and although Danny was still wheezing that night, when he woke up the next day, it was gone. This has never happened before! If Danny started wheezing, it usually lasted at least a week or two, and he would take so much medicine that he didn't sleep well and was very hard to live with.

Danny was also hyperactive and had difficulty in school doing his work and getting along with friends. I had him tested for Attention Deficit Disorder and was told he had slight Attention Deficit Order and Hyper-activity. They wanted to put him on Ritilin if it didn't improve. I am against any drugs and didn't want that to happen in any case.

Since we've been going to the chiropractor, his teacher has noticed many changes—an improvement in his ability to do his work and his coloring, and his general happiness because he feels better. His marks have improved in every subject on his report cards in school and in Hebrew school. He feels better about himself and hasn't had one puff on his inhaler since our first visit with the chiropractor.

Now my whole family sees the chiropractor. My daughter was told she had slight scoliosis and was just going to be watched by the orthopedic

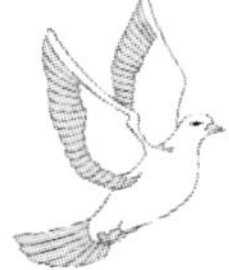

doctor. Since she has been adjusted by the chiropractor, she is walking straighter.

I've had a neck injury from whiplash for at least ten years and have constant pain in my ear. I've been through surgery and to several ear, nose and throat specialists. Nobody could help me. The chiropractor told me it will take at least five months to feel completely better, but I've already started to feel less pain. I lived on Advil in the past but haven't had to take it more than once or twice since seeing the chiropractor.

My husband also started going to the chiropractor. He was very reluctant at first because he had broken two vertebrae. He was afraid it would make him worse, but now he doesn't wake up in pain every morning. He has had more movement with his back than ever before. We're all thankful to Chiropractic for improving our health so much in such a short time!

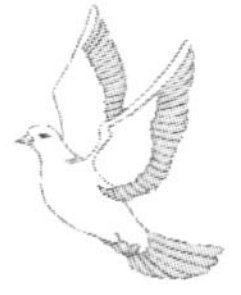

DAVID'S STORY • *David's Mother*

He was the most beautiful person I had ever seen. His huge blue eyes would stare up at me lovingly and his long lashes would brush his cheeks as he blinked. He fit perfectly into the crook of my arm and I could sit for hours just cuddling him. David was my first child, and he was the light of my life.

I had a relatively normal pregnancy. My first month had been torture with violent nausea and vomiting, then my obstetrician gave me a drug to control this problem. After the fourth month my nausea was gone and I no longer needed the drug. About three and a half weeks before my due date, my water broke. I did not go into labor so the next day it was induced. X-rays showed that the baby was not in position for birthing. My doctor turned him, and I had a natural vaginal delivery. David was born Friday, January 28, 1978, and as the nursery rhyme said about Friday's child, he was "loving and giving."

When David was six months old, he started having bouts of upper respiratory infections. They quickly progressed to the croup. His fevers would soar, and his cough was very dry and hacking. His breathing sounded so labored, and his intake of air sounded like he was gasping for his last breath. His pediatrician gave him antibiotics and warned me that the night time was the most critical time for him. The doctor said that the fever would go up and I would have to listen for any negative change in his breathing. If this

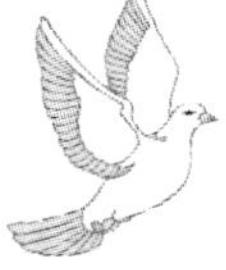

occurred, I was to immediately rush him to the hospital. On those nights I would camp out on the floor of David's bedroom listening to his every breath. Needless to say, I rarely slept and thanks to the humidifier, I felt like I was in the middle of a tropical rain forest.

David always recovered, and I marveled at the wonders of drugs and the brilliancy of the pediatrician. The only problem was that David kept getting sick and his bouts were lasting longer and getting worse. He went from the croup to ear infections and then to tonsillitis. By the time David was five years old, he was getting sick every three weeks just like clock work. He would sustain fevers of 106 degrees and would suffer from tonsillitis and severe stomach pains. These bouts now lasted for about a week and a half. His body looked like a pin cushion from all the needles the pediatrician gave him and he would suffer horribly with diarrhea and cramping from all the antibiotics. Added to this, he would dehydrate and have to spend days in the hospital hooked up to an I.V. His tonsils were always so swollen that they appeared to touch each other and even when he was "well" there were pus dots all over his tonsils. His colour was very pale. When he wasn't on antibiotics it was almost impossible for him to move his bowels. His once beautiful blue eyes were sunken and glassy. Dark circles were testimony to his sleepless nights and also to mine.

Because of David's constant sickness, he had missed most of his preschool classes and was in

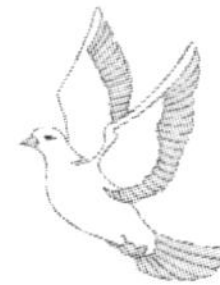

danger of having to repeat kindergarten. The pediatrician felt that there was nothing more that he could do for him and referred me to an ear, nose and throat specialist. This new doctor recommended surgery: removal of his adenoids and tonsils, tubes placed in his ears for proper drainage and something for his stomach which was always sour from draining pus. Surgery dates were set, and I prayed that David would stay well enough to have the operations because they could not be performed if he was sick.

Mothers of sick children have little time for pleasure, and something as insignificant as an hour away from their duties and a cup of coffee sounds like heaven to them. When my friend called me and invited me to come to a lecture being given by her new employer, a chiropractor, I hesitated. But, when she added the offer of coffee afterwards, I jumped at the suggestion. Fortunately, David was between bouts of tonsillitis and I met her at the doctor's office. I didn't hold much faith in Chiropractic but I decided to go with an open mind, not sure what to expect.

To my amazement, this man was the first person to explain to me why David was sick. He talked about wellness and health not just about disease.

He gave me hope and an understanding about how the human body works. I never got my coffee that night. I stayed after the lecture and bombarded the doctor with questions about my son. He answered them all and made me feel that there was nothing else he would rather

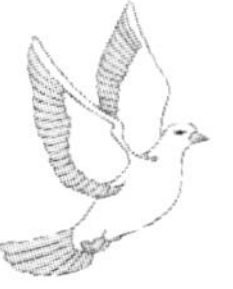

be doing. I came back to his office for a second lecture and brought with me a page full of new questions to ask him. He took all the time I needed to answer them, and in April I brought David in for an exam.

I was unused to the doctor's thoroughness and his willingness to take the time to explain all that was going on with David. His examinations found David to be suffering from malnutrition along with his many other symptoms. The mega-doses of various antibiotics had killed off the digestive bacteria's ability to process his food. That explained his suffering with constipation. David received Chiropractic adjustments three times a week and took herbal supplements to assist his body in healing itself. He did experience a few more bouts with tonsillitis, but each one was less severe than the one before, as predicted by the doctor.

In August, only four months after his first adjustment, David had his last tonsillitis attack. It lasted him only one day. He had a 99-degree temperature and there was only one tiny white dot on his tonsils. His day was spent playing on the beach, and he woke up feeling fine the next morning.

David just turned 18 last month. He's still one of the most beautiful people I have ever seen, full of life, love and creativity. He never did undergo the operations the specialists recommended, and had perfect attendance in first grade. The only explanation his pediatrician could give me about his seemingly

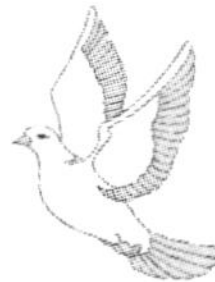

miraculous recovery was that he had outgrown his problems. We think not.

Chiropractic helped David reach a state of well-being that medicine can only be envious and jealous of. David now plays the base in a band and socializes with young people who call themselves "straight edge." They don't drink or smoke, and they DON'T DO DRUGS.

And now when David doesn't feel well he tells me, "Don't worry Mom, I just need an adjustment."

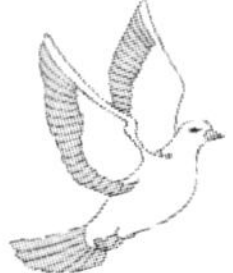

DEAFNESS • *Mrs. Olga Cribb*

It is a genuine pleasure to tell the world that Chiropractic caused a deaf person like me to be able to hear again. I threw away my hearing aid. For three years I had been deaf. I tried my family medical doctor, specialists, and even the Medical Center Hospital in Charleston. It cost me all my money and did nothing for my hearing. Can you imagine how it feels to go to church and not be able to hear the singing and preaching? To walk in the woods and not hear the birds or the wind blowing through the trees? It is a horrible and scary feeling of being alone.

Many of my relatives urged me to see a chiropractor. They had spoken so highly of their results that I decided to try for myself. The chiropractor found that a nerve was pinched causing me to be deaf. After a few adjustments my head felt clearer. In two weeks my hearing improved slightly. Little by little my hearing was completely restored three months after the first visit to the chiropractor.

No words can express my appreciation for Chiropractic. I have seen so many people get well since my first visit to the chiropractor. I think it is just wonderful how the chiropractor helps so many people.

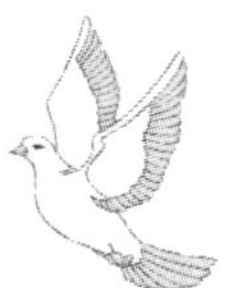

DEGENERATIVE DISCS • *Alison Theil*

I was diagnosed with Degenerative Disc Disease in 1987. For the past five years I have been getting by with pain killers and muscle relaxants. It became a daily part of my life.

In September, 1992, I had what I considered the worst attack I ever had. After numerous tests and X-rays, I was told that the doctors didn't know where my pain was coming from. They couldn't help me. For me that meant a continuation of pain killers and possibly the use of a cane to help me walk. I was out of work so much that I was on the verge of losing my job. I started to become very depressed.

Some very dear friends asked me if I would consider going to a chiropractor. I decided to give it a try.

I went to Dr. S. in November 1992. After reviewing my extensive collection of X-rays, Dr. S. told me that he could help me. I started receiving treatment four days a week. After two months of treatment with Dr. S., I could not believe the change in how I felt. I wanted to do the things I wasn't able to do for the last five years.

I have been coming to Dr. S. for 13 months now, my weight is down 25 pounds. This past summer I was able to start riding a bicycle as part of my therapy. I am now completely off pain killers. My energy level is much higher, and my outlook on the future is very positive.

I look back over the last six years and wonder how I lived with all that pain.

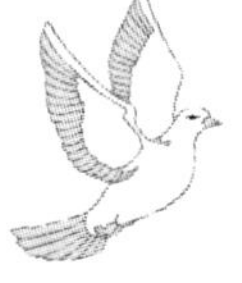

DIABETES • *Natalie K. Raw*

According to my doctors, I have four physical conditions that will require life-long care and treatment. The first condition is asthma, for which I get prescriptions for medication. The second condition is high blood pressure, for which I get prescriptions for medication. The third condition is diabetes, for which I get prescriptions for medication. The doctor can only give me pain pills for symptomatic relief, which I don't want because they are addictive. I frequently use a cane, and for a time I had to use a wheelchair.

In September, 1988, I went to the chiropractor in great pain, barely able to walk. In the four months that he has been treating me, he accomplished the following: I no longer use a cane, I am not in pain, I do not walk bent forward and to the right. There were times in the past that I could barely walk around the house. Now I can walk two miles and am working toward walking three miles. My blood pressure is down and the asthma is better.

The other big improvement is the diabetes. By adjusting my mid-back, where a nerve rod comes out that services the pancreas, he has been able to improve function and insulin production. My fasting blood sugar had gone from 230 to 84, a phenomenal decrease, and my medication has been adjusted appropriately. The chiropractor and I are working to get me off medication completely, and hopefully I will have

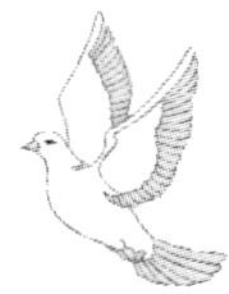

success with diet control.

The doctors diagnose my conditions and prescribe pills to take for the rest of my life for symptomatic relief. My chiropractor diagnoses my condition and works very hard on my behalf to improve the problem areas and get me off the pills.

The chiropractor has done more in four months to improve my physical self than a pulmonary specialist, an orthopedist and an internist had done in years.

Because my discovery of the chiropractor's expertise has benefited me to such a great degree, I wish to continue having him treat me. I look forward to continuing improvement in my health.

DOWN'S SYNDROME • *Bonnie Wells*

Karen was born February 23, 1969, and was diagnosed with Down's Syndrome. Karen has been through a lot in the early years of her life. For example, at 11 months old they told us she was going blind due to complications of glaucoma. By the time Karen was seven years old, she was fitted with two glass eyes. Besides the blindness, Karen was born with a major heart problem. She has a hole in the center of her heart that involves all four chambers. At her birth, I was told Karen would not live to be six years old because of her heart condition. The doctors also told me Karen would always be in and out of hospitals due to various illnesses and they were right.

At least two to three times a year she was in the hospital with pneumonia. Her lungs are so scarred they can not tell from X-rays if she has pneumonia anymore. Each time she would get sick they would give her antibiotics which would help her get well, but they also told me that eventually she would be immune to all of them and nothing would help her. Thank God, they were wrong!

In August 1985 we moved to Atlanta, Georgia. I went to a chiropractor in 1986 because of a back problem I was having. Chiropractic helped the pain in my back, but more than that, I learned that chiropractors are not pain doctors, but nerve doctors.

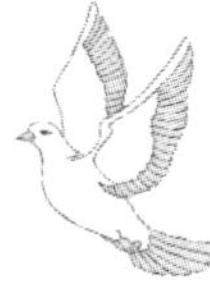

I also learned how Chiropractic can help many other symptoms and conditions, such as asthma, high blood pressure, lung problems, etc. ... as long as they are nerve related. I felt I had nothing to lose and everything to gain to have Karen examined. Dr. Pizza X-rayed Karen's cervical spine and found that she had a deformed atlas which is the top bone in the spine. That was the main reason that Karen held her head down all the time. The medical doctors told me she did it because of her blindness and she felt closer to the ground and more secure by doing that. Dr. Pizza explained to me that the nerves from the atlas bone go directly to the heart and lungs, and by getting her adjusted it would help her heart and lungs. It would also build her immune system up again. I agreed to start getting her adjusted. Well, that was ten years ago, Karen has not been in the hospital nor taken so much as an aspirin in those ten years.

Since that first adjustment, I started working for Dr. Pizza and now am starting my tenth year with him. Karen is now twenty-seven years old and has proved the medical profession wrong by getting better with Chiropractic. She has lived a lot longer than they said she would.

Chiropractic works and that's what counts!

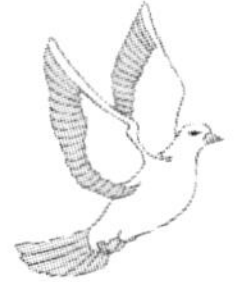

EAR INFECTIONS • *Margaret Sparks*

My daughter Natalie was suffering with severe ear infections or "Otitis Media." Natalie had this condition since she was three months old.

All that could be done for Natalie was to place her on antibiotics for a period of ten to fourteen days. Her ears would be clear for a period of a week or so, and then she would get another ear infection. This went on until she was about seventeen months old. By this time the doctors suggested tubes for her ears so her ears would drain correctly. I could not go along with this at all.

When I became an employee of Henry Chiropractic Clinic, I spoke to Dr. Henry about Natalie's problem. He said she could be helped through spinal adjustments to relieve the pressure and help her ears drain the fluid.

Natalie was given a spinal examination. Dr. Henry found tenderness in the area on her right side, which was always the most infected ear. Dr. Henry placed Natalie on an intensive care program with a vitamin supplement to build up her system to fight infections.

Natalie has changed so much. She is so full of life and is always up to something. She loves the outdoors and follows her older brother, trying to do whatever he is doing.

My friend Maurice received great relief when the chiropractor treated him for back problems that developed because of his long-

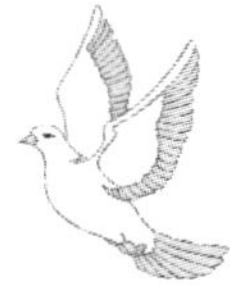

term desk job. My friend Hanne and her children were healed from various conditions (including recurring ear infections of her young daughter) as patients of Chiropractic. In fact, our chiropractor is the one health professional that I have never hesitated to recommend to friends and acquaintances.

Honestly, I almost always hesitate to recommend any form of therapy or any doctor to anyone, but I can easily say that this has not been true with Chiropractic. It is easy to mention this to anyone seeking health care because I can always trust they will get excellent treatment and positive health benefits.

I just remembered a time when the chiropractor treated my neck. He realized from examining my neck that I had a burning pain in my left calf, which I had not mentioned. After the treatment, all pain was gone.

The chiropractor always seems to know when a condition is in the realm of Chiropractic care. He treats such conditions with scientific precision. It is more than that. He is really a gifted healer with Chiropractic skills.

In this season of Thanksgiving, it is nice to remember the gifts and benefits we have received from others. In this case, I sincerely enjoy remembering the gifts of health that Chiropractic has brought us.

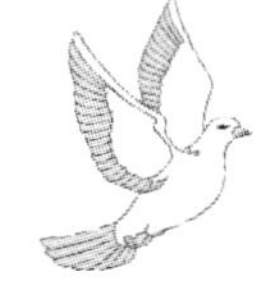

EAR INFECTIONS • *G. Thomas Kovacs, D.C.*

A four-and-a -half-year-old female was first brought to our office on January 9, 1995, for evaluation of chronic ear infections, a 50% right ear hearing loss, adenoiditis and asthma.

Medical History

The child was hospitalized at eight weeks with viral meningitis for three days, given medication via I.V. until veins collapsed, then medication was given via intra-muscular injection. Two weeks later the first of many ear infections with concomitant strep throat appeared. This condition continued on and off for four years, with only slight relief with medication during June, July and August.

In September 1994 she developed an ear infection which turned into bronchitis. Ceclor (oral antibiotic) was prescribed for 10 days. Two days following completion of Ceclor, she was put on Ceclor again, for another 10 days. Two days later a fever of 102 degrees developed. She was sent for a chest X-ray and was diagnosed as having pneumonia in both lungs. She was given Ceclor again in conjunction with Albuterol (a bronchodilator, not approved by FDA for children under 12) and a nebulizer: Ventolin and Intal (a bronchodilator and anti-inflammatory for asthmatics, respectively) for 20 days. The nebulizer and Albuterol were continued for one month.

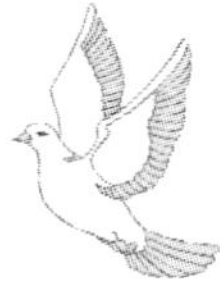

The child was also prescribed Pediapred (a steroid). On Thanksgiving Day she developed another ear infection, once again Ceclor was prescribed. In December she was given a flu shot and in two days developed croup. She was rushed to hospital, advised to stay on Ceclor and was also given a decongestant. On an airplane to Florida, the child had excruciating pain. A medical doctor at Disneyland prescribed Augmentin (an oral antibacterial/antibiotic) and Cardec-S syrup.

When the family returned home, a pulmonologist prescribed inhalers: Vanceril, Tilade and Proventil, all of which the child refused to take. He then prescribed Ventolin, Nasalide (a steroid) and Intal. The child was then referred to an ENT specialist who diagnosed enlarged adenoids, a 50% hearing loss and an inner ear infection. Surgery to remove the child's adenoids and to put tubes in her ears was scheduled.

Chiropractic History

On January 9, 1995, I examined the child chiropractically and found vertebral subluxations in her neck (cervical spine) and upper back (thoracic spine). A right sacroiliac (hip) subluxation was also found. Palpation of her neck revealed numerous enlarged lymph nodes and muscle spasm. The child was quite lethargic during the examination.

An Initial Intensive Phase of care of two times per week for six weeks was recommended. Dietary changes of decreased dairy and

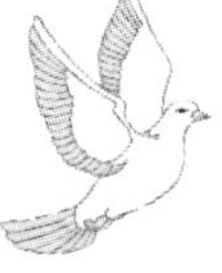

elimination of sugar was recommended, but not consistently adhered to. During Chiropractic care, subluxation patterns were very inconsistent and at first I questioned my findings. After three or four adjustments her mother noticed "a changed child, she has life in her body again." She stated that she started taking dance classes and "was acting like a little girl again for the first time in four years."

The major areas of involvement that I focused on were the 2nd cervical, 3rd thoracic and her right sacroiliac joint. However, other areas were involved at times. Light contacts and adjustments as taught by the ICPA pediatric program were delivered. I also utilized lymphatic and sinus drainage techniques on the child's head and neck.

After six weeks of Chiropractic care, a follow-up visit was made to her pediatrician and ENT specialist. Not only was there absolutely no sign of ear infection or inflammation, her adenoids, which were the worst the ENT had ever seen, were perfectly normal and healthy. Hearing tests revealed no hearing loss whatsoever. When the family was asked how long the child was on antibiotics, her family responded by saying "all medication was stopped six weeks ago when Chiropractic care started."

Shocked and confused by this answer, the family was told to continue Chiropractic care because it had obviously worked. The child is getting adjusted on a maintenance basis.

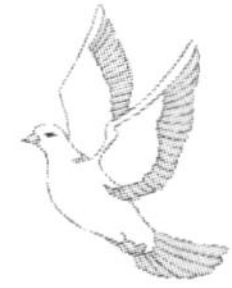

EPSTEIN BARR VIRUS • *Cathy Roberts*

I am 44 years old. I first came in to see Dr. Patzer because I had a pain down the side of one leg. Before starting treatment, I had been diagnosed with Epstein-Barr virus, chronic fatigue, allergy symptoms, hypothyroidism and depression. I have spent over $2,000 this year trying to find out why I feel so bad and keep getting worse.

I suffered from debilitating headaches, extreme fatigues, poor circulation in hands and feet, numbness in my toes, sore throats, sinus problems, herpes simplex, acne, short term memory loss, worsening eyesight, menstrual cramps, trouble maintaining attentiveness and a general feeling of losing control of my health.

Within the first month of Chiropractic treatment, I no longer suffer from the above. Hopefully, by the end of my active treatment, I will be able to quit taking medication for depression, hypothyroidism, and Epstein-Barr. I hope that my eyesight and memory loss will no longer be a problem.

I feel so much better about my life and my future. Believe it or not, I am so thankful for that pain in my leg. If not for that pain, I would never have discovered that I had brain stem damage and several subluxations in my spine. I would never have learned the important part your spine plays in your entire life.

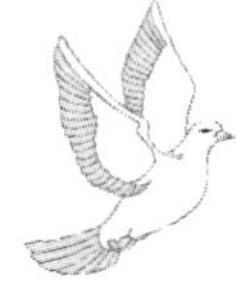

EMPHYSEMA • *Jo Ann Gengopoulos*

I like to think of myself as a happy-go-lucky personality type. I am very out-going and have been told all my life that I am disgustingly over optimistic. It's very difficult to keep up an image like this when you don't feel well.

For four long years I have been under constant treatment. I have three specialists taking care of me and I have a medical history about three inches thick, with no exaggeration. I have been diagnosed with emphysema, asthma, severe allergies, PID (pelvic inflammatory disease), IBS (irritable bowel syndrome), a hormone disorder, a nervous disorder and a hemorrhoid problem that required two laser surgeries. Neither of these surgeries helped my situation.

I have been prescribed medication that is phenomenal—from Atrovent inhaler to Xanax, which is a tranquilizer. Through all of these prescriptions, I never felt better, and I could not understand why I was always sick and in so much pain. Because of all the medications I have been taking, I now have very weak veins and a duodenal ulcer.

On February 13 my back went out. I was afraid to seek Chiropractic care because I was so tired of going to doctors. On February 1 my OB/GYN scheduled a hysterectomy for the beginning of April. Naturally I had the attitude like: "What else is going to happen to me?" On

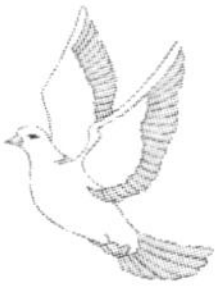

February 16 I came into the Chiropractic clinic. I came here because in the beginning of this year my husband came in. He has recuperated well.

At the time I was not only experiencing severe back pain, but also pain in my lower abdomen for which I was taking Vicoden ES, but the pain would not go away. After my first adjustment, the pain in my lower abdomen was completely gone. My back did feel much better, but naturally it did bother me.

I couldn't believe it! I was afraid to say anything about this particular pain stopping because I thought the doctor would think I was nuts.

In 1992, I spent just short of $70,000 in hospital bills and $6,200 in prescriptions. I had cryosurgery, colonoscopy, laparotomy, two laparoscopies, two laser surgeries, Barium enemas, Barium swallows, and numerous X-rays and sonograms. Last year I was also given Lupron, which is an experimental medication which costs $375 per injection every three weeks for six months. Nothing, and I mean nothing, helped me. UNTIL ... two weeks ago. I am feeling much better and I have not taken one single pill since then.

It's a terrible thing when you go to a medical doctor for help and all they do is pull out that Rx pad and start writing. I am not saying that they are uncaring and callous; it's just that they do not believe the possibilities of nerves controlling the functional rhythms of the human body.

All I can say is Thank God my back went

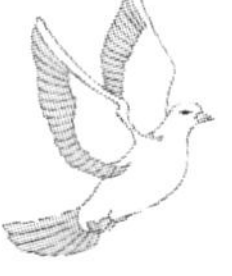

out when it did, otherwise I would have had that hysterectomy for nothing. It will take time to get my body to normal after all the medication I have been on, but anything is better than the way I was.

After all this time of walking through a dark tunnel of pain and agony, I now see a light. It is ironic to think that I could have saved myself all this pain and suffering if I had my back checked a long time ago when I first had back problems. This was the root of all my so-called medical disorders.

Thanks for Chiropractic care!

The following is the medication I was taking – although, I couldn't remember them all:

Amoxicillin 500mg		Dioxycyclene	Lupron
Seldane,	Axid	Erythromycin	Orudis
Tetracycline	Buspar	Procto Cream	Esgic
Tylenol #3	Ceclor	Fioricet	Reglan
Tylenol #4	Compazine	Flexeril	Runatan
Vibramycin	Darvocet-N	Ibuprofen 800 mg	Sardol
Vicodin	Vicodin ES	Xanax	Atrovent

Too many prescriptions for one body to take.

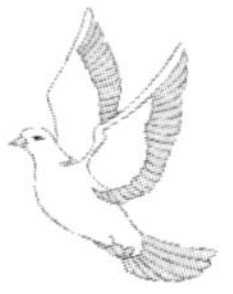

ENLARGED LIVER

• *Joseph A. LaBarbera, D.C.*

Even after practicing for seven years I am still astonished at the results achieved utilizing Chiropractic care on sick patients. I am not referring to the back aches and stiff necks, but rather to those individuals with altered physiology and dis-ease in their body. Mike D. was one of these individuals. He was first seen on July 14, 1992, on the referral of another patient.

Mike is a 47-year-old man with a multitude of complaints. He came into my office with a stoppage gait, slapping each foot down as he moved forward. He staggered and was very unsteady when he ambulated. He stated that he was unable to feel anything below his knees and that he had very little strength in his legs. This condition came on gradually a month earlier and was worsening each day. Until this time he was a cable splicer for NY Telephone; now he could hardly care for himself.

Before being seen by me, he had been through the typical medical route. A CT scan of the abdomen showed an enlarged liver. Blood chemistries revealed altered liver enzymes. After many tests and evaluations by specialists throughout the area, a diagnosis of "Alcohol Induced Neuropathy" was made. He was told nothing could be done for him and that he should make plans to be in a nursing home by December. He was told to prepare himself for a liver transplant by the spring. It was

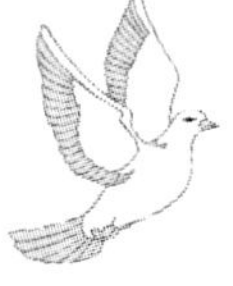

recommended that he stop drinking all alcohol and to discontinue smoking. A physical therapy treatment was established for him.

My evaluation of Mike showed complete loss of bilateral lower extremity reflexes even with reinforcement, inability to heel walk and a +3 Toe walk bilaterally. All other Ortho-Neuro exams were essentially negative. X-ray analysis revealed an upper cervical subluxation complex involving Atlas and Axis. There were other misalignments in the cervical and limbo-pelvic spine, but due to the severity of his symptoms, I decided to apply strictly Knee/Chest/Upper Cervical Specific adjusting procedures. This includes monitoring utilizing the Thermoscribe II (neurocalometer).

Working totally outside any guidelines set forth by individual groups or IME recommendations, I cared for Mike on a routine basis for the following seven months. In that time frame he had numerous falls and broken toes due to his condition. Many visits consisted of only a scan and no adjustment (he still had symptoms). He was determined to get well and followed my advice to the letter. Gradual improvements were seen, subtle at first.

He began to wiggle his toes and then his feet. Sensation and then strength came back. He started walking for exercise every two weeks now and was adjusted about once per month. His liver was checked and coincidentally returned to normal size and his enzymes stabilized. Mike still has a beer and cigarette, but with the "power of the innate" on the job,

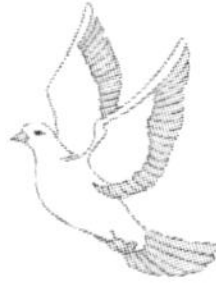

he is able to handle the toxic effects. He is looking forward to returning to work and living life to the fullest.

This case shows the dramatic effect Chiropractic care can have on someone so far gone. What effects can it have on someone apparently healthy? The bottom line is to care for your patients as if their lives depend on it, because they do. I know Mike is ecstatic for the existence of Chiropractic. Each time I see him I am reminded about the unlimited powers of innate. It is up each doctor to release it.

ENLARGED LIVER • *Pam Nelson*

Dear Dr. John and Sue,

I have been wanting to write this for a long time.

I want to thank you for the good health I am experiencing because it has changed my life. Your care over the past two and a half years has brought about a gradual, but steady improvement that has literally given me quality health. It sounds clinical and blasé on paper, however, the meaning touches a deeper chord than I can express.

When you are in chronic pain, you lose the ability to do simple everyday tasks. You miss activities that bring pleasure. You aren't productive. The focus of your life is simply trying to survive.

I was suffering on an emotional level as well because my health burdened my family, and the fear of what was happening to me was devastating. When the focus in your life is pain and fear, you lose much more than the obvious; you lose hope and optimism that motivates us to achieve happiness.

Prior to seeing you, I had some very negative experiences with doctors. The last experience was so bad I was afraid to seek any help whatsoever and unable to trust any doctor's judgment. I had symptoms such as severe headaches, dizziness, nausea, stiff neck, ear ache, that were increasing. I was given antibiotics, injections and

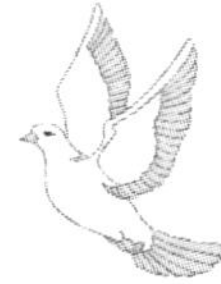

pills, and was diagnosed with sinus and inner ear infection.

After several more visits I was given yet more antibiotics plus a prescription for pills for dizziness. Let me add here that the side effect of that prescription was dizziness! I kept telling the medical doctor that I'd had a "bad back," I felt "out of balance." He insisted none of these could possibly have any bearing on an infection of the inner ear and sinuses.

Within a short time I was rushed to the hospital emergency room. My liver was enlarged and not functioning properly. I'd told the doctors about the many injections and antibiotics I'd had, as well as the back and teeth complaints.

They said all that was irrelevant. After numerous tests all that was indicated was the liver malfunctioning—no sign of infection at all. Yet the symptoms I'd been treated for initially persisted. Since they couldn't diagnose what caused the radical liver condition, they persisted to ask if I was a heavy alcohol drinker. I have never even been an occasional drinker.

Whenever I'd mention the many recent prescriptions of antibiotics in heavy dosages, I was ignored and "hushed." The prescribing doctor came to the hospital and had a conference with the hospital staff. He showed more concern then. The liver specialist and hospital staff doctors ran battalions of tests and kept me on an I.V. solution because my liver couldn't filter toxins. They insisted I must drink alcohol because there was no disease present to cause this kind of liver reaction. Basically, my liver had

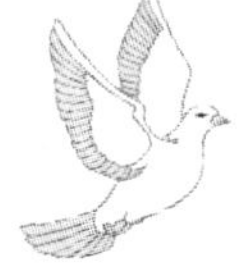

been overwhelmed with something. So, I was released and given Fiorinol for headaches, muscle relaxants for neck pain, and an antibiotic in case the non-existent infection persisted!

The next three months I continued to see the specialist until my liver was functioning and I was able to sleep less than 20 hours a day. When I came home I threw out the medication because I knew it was the culprit, I'd been overdosed with antibiotics I did not need and my body was reacting to the toxic effect. The end diagnosis was a "virus," yet the tests and records never revealed this.

I was a victim, a lucky victim, of our society's addiction to "a quick fix" through prescribing harmful and often unnecessary drugs to treat symptoms. This cycle causes a lot of harm; not only does it prevent looking for underlying problems that are "screaming" for attention through symptoms, but it creates many conditions aside from that.

If half the attention given to my liver's reaction to drugs had been applied to finding the source of the symptoms ... well, I'd never have had a liver problem in the first place. It was a traumatic experience that caused a lot of pain and three months to recover. My original symptoms increased in severity until I couldn't turn my head or walk; the headaches and dizziness made me feel "crazy" and the earache and nausea prevented appetite, etc.

At this point I came to a chiropractor's office. It was an ordeal to ride in the car, to maintain balance and seem "coherent." At that

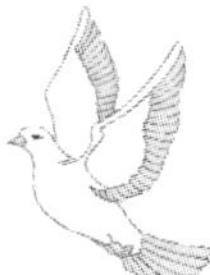

time I was afraid to accept or believe or trust any medical philosophy, but I knew chiropractors would not prescribe drugs and that was my comfort! It was scary to trust adjustments because as severe as my symptoms were, I was convinced I had a serious ailment that was being neglected. I had several months of frequent adjustments without feeling much better.

Those first months I relied on adjustments ranging from twice a day to every day to several times a week, just to control pain. As I began to "last" longer between adjustments and the symptoms lessened in severity and frequency, I began to believe and have faith in Chiropractic. It's hard to doubt the reality of what you feel! It becomes difficult to ignore the obvious, though, when you experience the benefits it brings. I've learned to take an active role in what I choose to allow for myself. We can all assume responsibility to make decisions on our own behalf, on behalf of our health.

We have been trained to reach for "quick fixes" to the point we destroy our body's own healing processes. We're too eager to intervene and interfere with a natural process.

It's reasonable to take an antibiotic when an infection is too advanced for our immune system to control it or if our immune system is diseased or unable to function on it's own. It is not reasonable to use antibiotics as prevention or before allowing our bodies to heal themselves. I left the hospital diagnosed with a virus and an antibiotic (how many times this has happened to me), yet an antibiotic kills bacteria not a virus.

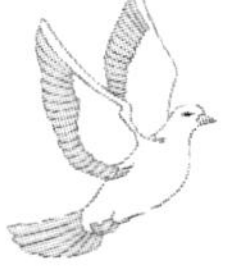

We need to question more the familiar routine route to medical care and be less skeptical of the natural alternatives that cause no harm.

After two and a half years of Chiropractic adjustments, I have seen incredible improvements in my health. NOT taking pain pills or antibiotics has allowed my immune system to function and do it's job. It is healthy and doesn't require intervention. I have not had an infection, a cold, or the flu since I've chosen adjustments over antibiotics. Without pain pills I can listen to my symptoms instead of masking them.

As you suggested, I am seeing a dentist who is "balancing" my occlusion (bite) to restore and replace missing teeth. This will correct an imbalance in jaw structure and allow upper vertebrae and cranial structures to sit in alignment. That problem alone caused fluid build-up in my ear (mimicking an infection) and prevented normal sinus functions. All the drug therapy in the world could only mask symptoms: it takes searching for underlying causes of symptoms to find answers.

Doctors did not want to look at why my back and neck hurt. They focused on tests to indicate which drugs to prescribe. I'm sorry, but I can't buy the theory that a chemical can adjust the spine or vertebrae to keep nerves functioning. I can't find any logic in muscle relaxants accomplishing what exercise and adjustments can do. My liver couldn't accept it either.

I've had many people warn me about Chiropractic. We're all aware of the negative scare tactics surrounding it. Who is telling us

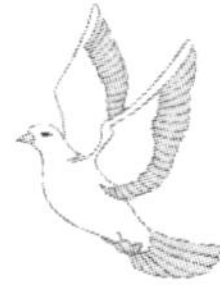

these things? The very doctors who are not doing us a beneficial service with their treatments and people who are not healthy or realizing benefits! I have never been advised against Chiropractic by anyone who is drug-free and healthy and reaping the good results. The reason seems to be because healthy, happy people don't share positive things, while we all tend to blab incessantly about pain and problems!

I've needed to let you all know how much you've helped me and how appreciative I am that you took the time to educate me about a healthier, more sensible way to improve my health. It is rare to find someone who is so devoted and committed to serving others and who believes it is important to leave this world a bit better than they found it. You are sincere and genuine in your philosophy. You use common sense and safe practices that have restored my health beyond what I thought was possible.

Chiropractic adjustments were a common-sense method of helping my body heal itself and function as it was meant to do. No drugs, no side effects, just time to heal and allowing Mother Nature to do what she does best. It is true, "the power that made the body, heals the body."

FEVERS • *D.S.*

November 20, 1984

I remembered some of the times you treated me, my son and some of my friends with such positive results. On one occasion, my two-year-old developed a sudden fever. I remembered that earlier that day a neighbor who had been watching him reported to me that he had fallen from a parked motorcycle. I immediately connected his symptoms with the fall and took him to your office right away. Sure enough, his fever and crankiness disappeared a short time after you treated him.

On another occasion I developed a pretty bad headache. I do not usually suffer from headaches. In a matter of minutes after my treatment all symptoms were relieved.

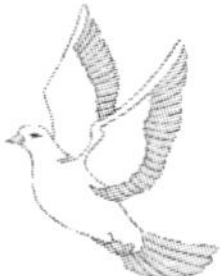

HEADACHES • *Mary Brault*

I found myself reluctantly seeking Chiropractic care in an attempt to get relief from severe migraine headaches. I had already seen many other doctors and had tried medications, from over the counter drugs to some very heavy prescription remedies. The only "miracle drug" that stopped the headaches was an injection that came with a whole set of side effects. I continued on this "road to recovery" and realized that the headaches were more frequent and more severe.

At this point I was desperate and could only hope that Chiropractic could help. What did I have to lose?

After my first adjustment I had increased mobility; looking freely from the right to the left without wincing through the pain was new to me. There have been other subtle but very welcome benefits. My energy levels have increased and the tension has been replaced by a new level of calm serenity. I have also shed unwanted pounds and sleepless nights are memories of the past. I find that my thoughts are more focused and less scattered. This is all most impressive since I have only had treatments for three weeks.

Without a doubt, the single most important benefit I have received from Chiropractic care is that I have found a form of treatment I feel comfortable with. This alternative feels so much better than a prescription for the latest drug of

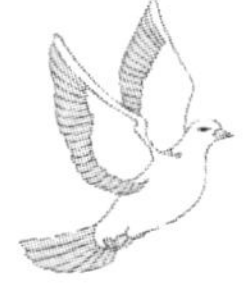

choice. There are enough quoted statistics of women that take hormone replacements drugs to take care of normal body changes. I'm finally asking some tough questions about my body and getting great answers.

At this point, I am not taking any prescriptions. For the first time in over five years, I'm getting relief from migraine headaches. I finally feel in tune with my body. In general, I'm feeling better than I have in a long time. Thanks to Chiropractic care!

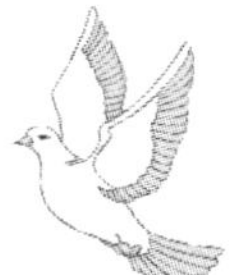

HEADACHES • *Patsy Cox*

It's a distinct pleasure to tell you what Chiropractic has done for me. For as long as I can remember my legs have given me a great deal of pain. Along with this, my back hurt constantly. About five years ago I started developing headaches. At first, simple headache remedies would give me relief, but after a while nothing would. In five years I tried six doctors. All gave me different medications, none of which helped. By this time my headaches were driving me crazy, and I was frantic for relief. After talking to some of my relatives who had been to a chiropractor, I decided to see if Chiropractic could help me.

The doctor took X-ray pictures of my entire spine and showed me the cause of my trouble. The first adjustment of my spine caused my headaches to leave immediately. Three or four days after this, my legs and back quit hurting. It has now been three months since the chiropractor first worked on me.

I can truly say it has been my healthiest three months. It seems silly for sick people to suffer when Chiropractic can help them.

HEADACHES • *Gladys Johnston*

My name is Gladys Johnson. For over 25 years I suffered with debilitating headaches that would last constantly for three to four weeks! During these headaches I was unable to work, I couldn't perform my routine household duties, and they made it difficult for me to function with my six children and eight grandchildren. My medical doctor gave me prescription after prescription, but nothing worked.

Over a period of time, I became friends with a lady who swore that a chiropractor would help me with my headaches without any medication! It took her a long time to convince me that someone other than a medical doctor could relieve my nasty headaches.

Well, after two months of a constant headache, I took her advice, and my life changed. I had one adjustment and my headache went away!

Since then I have been under care for nine months and I can count the number of headaches I have had on one hand! My outlook on life has changed, my energy level has increased. My family is much happier now that I don't complain of headaches. Chiropractic has changed my life! For that, I am grateful.

Thank you!

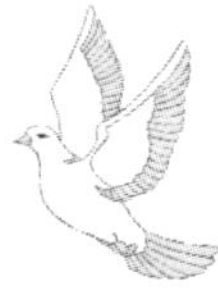

HEARING LOSS

• *Kelly, Raymond and Matthew Rizzo*

Dear Dr. Goldfarb,

Where do we begin to thank you for how you've touched our lives? When we came to you with Matthew's problem, I'll be honest in saying, we were not sure how a chiropractor was going to be able to help an infant's hearing problem. After going from ear doctor to ear doctor, all the results were coming out the same, that Matthew, our six month old son, had a hearing loss that would require surgery and hearing aides, probably for life. Then someone suggested that we see a Chiropractor. I thought it was a little strange taking a baby to a chiropractor, but we were willing to try anything to help him.

Well, to our amazement that same night after you examined and treated Matthew, he was hearing sounds. He woke up when hearing the doors lock on the car and again when crumpling a bag. Within a few days we were convinced he was hearing just fine. One week later, we took him to an ear specialist in Manhattan. He found Matthew's hearing to be 100% normal. They cancelled the surgery and were amazed at the sudden change.

I believe Matthew hears better than any one of us. So, we thank you, Dr. Goldfarb for helping us with your miracle hands. We are so glad you were able to help us and we know this will leave a lasting impression on all our lives.

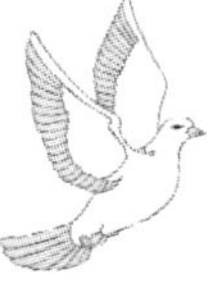

HEART PAIN • *Agostino Aliberti*

I want to thank you for the help that you are giving me. You have changed my life.

I have been to so many doctors in the past year and taken just about every medication you can think of. I had just about given up. I thought to myself: I'm only 34 years old, and I feel like my life is over because of the physical pain I was having and the weird symptoms I had prior to coming to you.

I was having not only pain in my heart area, but palpitations and numbness in my hands and my hand would shake. My social life was at a stand still. I was at my wits' end.

You have given me some relief already, and I know with your continued help that I'll become a normal person again and resume my life.

Thank you so much!

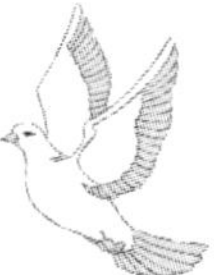

HEMORRHOIDS • *James A. Lowe*

One morning I woke up with the most awful pain a human could experience. I had heard about it, I had read about it, I had heard it whispered about, and now I was having it. I was having an attack of horrible, hurting hemorrhoids. The pain was so bad I couldn't sit, walk or work. I tried everything that was sold, invented or advertised that was said to be good for hemorrhoids. The results were nothing, except more pain.

One day I went with my wife to visit her chiropractor. While the doctor was treating her, I asked him if Chiropractic could help hemorrhoids. To my surprise he said, "Yes," and told me that lots of people come with that problem. I told him if he could fix me, "Please get started."

If it hadn't happened to me, I would have found it hard to believe. The doctor adjusted my lower spine, and the next morning I was fifty percent better. In three days all the pain and swelling left and I could sit in comfort on a hard chair. I can honestly say they're gone! They're gone! My hemorrhoids are gone! This surely has made a believer out of me.

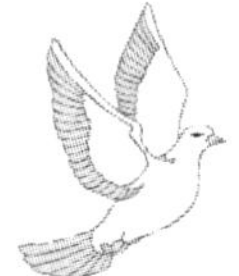

I DON'T BELIEVE IN CHIROPRACTIC

• *Mel Barlin*

I didn't believe in Chiropractic!

I took my son David to see Doctor P. in July for chronic back pain, out of desperation. He'd been suffering for several years. The doctor X-rayed David and told him, "David, you have a lot of neck pain, too." David said, "How did you know?"

In two months both the back and neck pain were virtually gone. Occasional twinges remind David to keep up his exercises.

Next came my wife. She sits in front of a computer all day. She has severe lower back problems. Thanks to Dr. P., the pain is going.

Then, kicking and screaming, came me. There was nothing wrong with me. After the X-ray the doctor asked me how long I've had plumbing problems. I said, "How did you know?" I'd been getting up to urinate four or five times a night. After ten weeks, thanks to Dr. P., I'm sleeping through the night.

When our other two kids come back from school this summer, we're taking them to our chiropractor, too.

We are now believers.

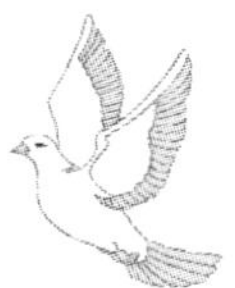

INFERTILITY

• *Donna M. Rickey*

June 6, 1990

It all started on August 8, 1989, with my fist visit to Dr. Wittner. I was experiencing a lot of lower back and abdominal pain for more than a year. I had been put through numerous tests by my regular physician. There were two kidney IVP Drip tests, and let me tell you, they were no fun. The dye they inject in you for the test makes you nauseous. In some cases people are allergic to the dye, and they get even more sick. After two gall bladder tests, they tried a pelvic ultrasound and an upper G. I. series. The next step for me was to go the hospital for an exploratory, but I stopped there.

I had never been to a chiropractor before, and I was a little skeptical about going, but I was willing to try any alternative at this point. This turned out to be the best decision that I could have made. The chiropractor's assistant asked me some personal questions regarding how long I had been married. She also asked if we had any children and if we wanted to have children. I proceeded to tell her that I had been married for over eight years and that we had no children. Art, my husband, had five children from his first marriage. I told her that we weren't using anything to prevent a pregnancy, but if it happened, we would be happy. If I didn't have any children, then that was what was meant to

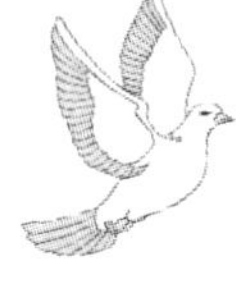

be. I was not going to be aggressive in discovering why I could not conceive. Carol then joked about it and said that maybe after Dr. Wittner did all his adjustments on me and got me back in good shape I would get pregnant. I asked her if she was serious, and she said that you could never know about these things; anything could possibly happen.

At this point Dr. Wittner came into the room, and we introduced ourselves to each other. He proceeded to ask me what my problem was and my medical history up to that point. I explained it to him, as I did before to Carol. He said he had a good understanding of my problem and wanted to examine my spine, but was not going to give me an adjustment that day. After he examined my spine, he then wanted to take a few X-rays, to have a better picture of my problem and to confirm his suspicion of what the problem was. He told me that he knew I did not have a life-threatening condition and that he was positive that he could help me.

Dolly explained that there was an open-door policy and that the only time that you need an appointment is if you are a new patient. I thought this was a great idca, and I left there feeling more relaxed then I had in a long time.

When I returned, after watching the very informative video, I was shown to one of the rooms and placed on the table. Dr. Wittner came in shortly thereafter. He explained that my problem was in the lumbar area of my spine:

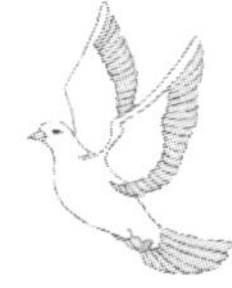

It was correctable and there was no sign of arthritis in my spine. He could not tell me how long or how many adjustments it would take to correct, but in time my problem would be gone.

He then said he would start giving me my adjustments. Dr. Wittner told me that I should only feel some pressure, but no pain. This certainly relaxed me because I did not know what to expect. After the adjustments, which only take a few minutes, Dr. Wittner asked to see me in the office. He explained that as my condition improved, my visits would be reduced.

I have to admit, I did feel good after my adjustments, and after a few visits I realized that I didn't know why it took me so long to find Chiropractic. Well, after all the adjustments I have had since August 8, I am feeling great. My persistent pain is gone. I did not have to have any surgery. I am now going once or twice a month for adjustments, and I feel fantastic.

The best news is yet to come. On May 8, 1990, I found out I was pregnant. After nine years of trying, I was finally going to have a baby. Both my husband and I are ecstatic. I believe in my heart, if I never started going to Dr. Wittner, I would not be pregnant now.

I would like to thank Dr. Wittner with all my heart for not only correcting my original problem, but for introducing me to the world of Chiropractic. Thank you again, Dr. Wittner.

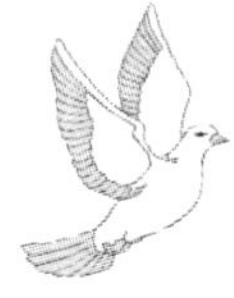

INJURY • *Ron's Story*

In January of 1991, I was stationed in Saudi Arabia during Desert Storm. I sustained an injury which caused quite a bit of pain in the lower shoulder blade area. I tried various forms of stretching and loosening exercises. I was eating Tylenol for breakfast, lunch and dinner.

My wife Gayle has been a Chiropractic patient since March 1991, and she suggested I make an appointment with her doctor.

I had a consultation with the chiropractor, an examination and X-rays. The X-rays showed a curvature of the spine. I was scheduled for a series of spinal manipulations and instructed on an exercise program.

I'm no longer in pain, and I can sleep again. I feel about 1000% better!

Try Chiropractic! You'll like it!

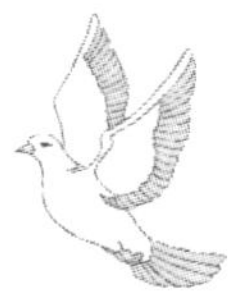

LEARNING DISABILITIES

• *Elana Brown, D.C.*

When Tabitha started school, she had speech problems and learning difficulties. We were told Tabitha did not have normal mental maturity, and she possibly had slight brain damage. Her birthing was difficult. She was a large baby weighing 10 pounds, 10 ounces (at birth). She did not pass to first grade.

Her hearing was tested, and the results showed no hearing problem. Three years of speech therapy showed little improvement. The learning disability specialists at school said Tabitha's low mental maturity was probably due to slight brain damage.

I was receiving Chiropractic treatments for an injury caused in a car accident. After speaking with the receptionist at the doctor's office about my daughter, she suggested I bring Tabitha in for a check-up.

The chiropractor examined her and took X-rays to see where the problem was. He started treatments, and I also worked with her. Tabitha's response to Chiropractic care has been remarkable. When we started treatments she knew four of the letters of the alphabet, since then there has been a rapid increase of letter recognition. She has a way to go, but has improved a lot. She is more attentive, alert and outgoing. Her teacher said there has been quite a change in her, and she has been promoted to first grade.

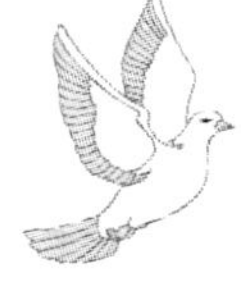

Give Chiropractic a try before accepting somebody's opinion that your child has a learning disability or any other kind of permanent disability.

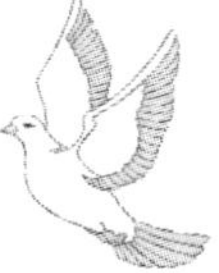

LUCKY ANTHONY • *Dr. Arthur Patterson Jr.*

Imagine you're a tiny baby.

You struggle every waking moment to take in a breath. Every week, for the first four years of your life, you are tortured by asthma attacks so severe that you must be hospitalized. Your life is an endless stream of emergency rooms, doctors, gasping for air, nausea and vomiting from side effects of the potent medications you are injected with or which you ingest each day with the hope of somehow rectifying your desperate situation. Four long years when your mother, aunt, teachers and friends did not know what to say or do to help you. Highly educated and revered doctors are helpless to assist you in your torment.

All the Proventil, Ventolin, Albuterol, Theodur, Prednisone has been prescribed to you with no avail. The other kids run around gleefully playing. All you can do is watch them, longingly.

This was the true, sad description of Anthony Caceres.

Until one day your Aunt Rosa heard a chiropractor on the radio discussing the unique science and art of Chiropractic. He seems more positive and upbeat than the endless line of clinics you've been dragged to with NO RESULTS, Aunt Rosa thought.

The family takes a chance. They give Chiropractic a try. LUCKY YOU! That was five years ago. You've never taken a drug again since

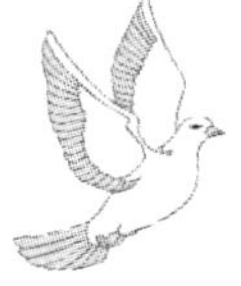

your first adjustment. It wasn't magic, but it worked. Every day for two years you went for your life enhancing, energy releasing, health restoring Chiropractic adjustment, drug free. In the first year you needed to go to the hospital once. Since then, you've never returned: drug free. For the first three years you still had attacks now and again, but never as severe as before. In the past two years you've only had three or four tough periods. NO attacks! The rest has been quite enjoyable.

After all, for someone who was robbed of every precious breath and filled with dangerous chemicals for the first four years of your life, Chiropractic is a welcome friend.

LYME DISEASE • *Mary Seaman*

Dear Doctor,

I just want to thank you for all you've done for my daughter Nicole. Two months ago I went to you out of desperation. As you recall, on our first visit I expressed my skepticism of Chiropractic care. Nicole was being treated for Lyme disease with high doses of antibiotics for nearly one year. Her symptoms were severe headaches, sore throat, painful and swollen joints, and chronic fatigue. She took pain pills every four hours to make it through her school day – which wasn't often.

It was heartbreaking to watch my little girl deteriorate before my eyes. I watched my daughter, who previously would go to dance class, play with her friends, ride her bike, and do all the other things kids do, come home and go to bed or lie on the couch instead. If I hadn't seen the miraculous improvement within weeks of your treatment, I never would have believed it.

She is now off all medication, with the exception of an occasional aspirin. She is back to dancing, playing and doing all the things a ten year old does. I can never express my gratitude or thank you enough for giving me back my little girl. I will never again doubt the importance and value of Chiropractic care.

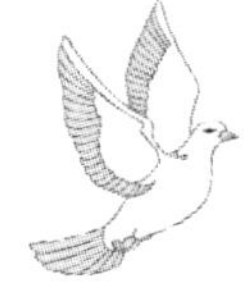

MANDY'S CURE • *Patricia S. Bruce*

On October 29, 1984, we had our first child, a beautiful, healthy baby girl. Mandy was only six weeks old when she was hospitalized for a life-threatening asthma attack. Between six weeks and 15 months she was hospitalized more times than I can remember. We traveled from one specialist to another under the recommendation of Mandy's pediatrician.

She had numerous procedures, allergy tests and other tests that we thought were necessary to help her overcome her asthma. Mandy had taken more medications in her first 12 months than most people take in a lifetime. She was not getting any better. They just helped her tolerate her frequent, severe asthma attacks.

As Mandy's asthma attacks continued, the medications were increased. We knew that pumping our child full of steroids and other drugs (while continuing to see her suffer with asthma and the mediations' side effects) was dangerous to her health. Mandy was on so many medications that we had to keep a written log of the type, dosage and time given. The medicine was causing her to have diarrhea, and she was vomiting constantly. She became hyperactive after certain medications and was hardly sleeping at all. Sedatives were prescribed.

The medical doctors told us not to be so concerned with the medications or their side effects because without them she could die.

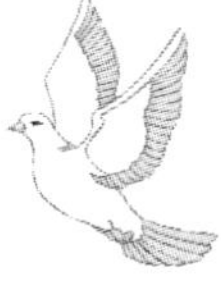

At this point we were sure we had to do something, but we had no idea of what to do. On numerous occasions we questioned the prescription and dosage prescribed for such a small baby. On one occasion the pharmacist was very reluctant to fill the prescription the doctor had written and called the doctor expressing his concern that it may have been written incorrectly. After the doctor confirmed what was written, the pharmacist returned with the medicine and he gave me a long brochure that he had on the medicine. He asked me to read it because he too was concerned that Mandy was being overmedicated. The pharmacist advised us to again confront Mandy's doctors with the information he had provided.

When I went to the doctor with my concerns and questions, he told me that without these drugs our daughter would die. We were devastated by the fact that Mandy needed these drugs to live. This is when we became more determined than ever to find a better way.

Shortly after Mandy was hospitalized in November 1986, I ran into an older lady that worked in a coffee shop in East Point. The last time I had seen her I was pregnant with Mandy. When she asked about my baby, I told her about her asthma and without hesitation she said, "Don't let that baby suffer another day. Take her to a chiropractor. I had asthma attacks for 50 years and can't recall having any attacks since I began seeing a chiropractor 10 years ago."

All day long I thought about what she said.

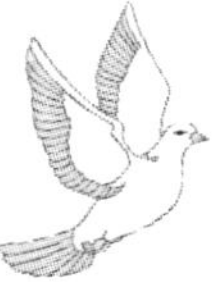

Later when I discussed it with Robert, he said, "Why not? We have tried everything else!" Initially we decided I would go first to see exactly what they did. I had back problems so that was the perfect reason to check one out. I found an ad in a local newspaper. At the time, I had no idea that the chiropractor would be Mandy's healer.

I made an appointment with the chiropractor that week because Mandy was sick and I did not want to waste any time in checking him out to see if he could help her. I knew nothing, I repeat, nothing at all about chiropractors, and I was very anxious when I arrived for my first visit. Everyone in the office was friendly and professional. I saw nothing in the chiropractor's office that I needed to be afraid of. The adjustment I received was painless. I still was not sure if he could help Mandy until I went to his doctor's report and realized that chiropractors wanted the same thing I did: a drug-free healthy body.

I felt comfortable enough to discuss Mandy with the chiropractor. He was genuinely concerned and wanted to see her immediately. Mandy saw the chiropractor three times a week. We immediately began to see a change in her. The chiropractor wanted Mandy off all drugs right away which is certainly what we wanted, but we were still not totally convinced.

She had been seeing several asthma specialists at SRCH for over a year and the chiropractor for only a few weeks. Prior to

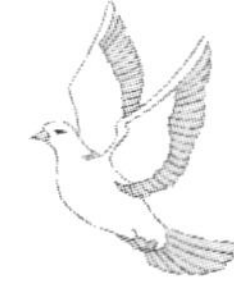

seeing the chiropractor, Mandy was scheduled for a larygnoscopy/bronchoscopy/tracheoscopy on February 20, 1986. The physicians we had been taking her to all agreed that her asthma was unusually bad and this diagnostic surgery was necessary to rule out tumors or other obstruction of the airway.

The chiropractor asked us not to put her through the surgery. He wanted us to give him a little more time with her. I regret my decision to this day.

Mandy's surgeon called us after it was over. In about two minutes he told us the surgery went well and there were no tumors or other abnormalities. Mandy had severe asthma. He also said she would need to stay on the medication continuously to avoid more life-threatening attacks.

The same afternoon Robert and I decided that we would put more faith in the chiropractor because he was the only doctor that could offer Mandy the results we wanted with NO DRUGS!

Because of the types of medications she was taking, we had to taper her off very gradually. We began this process the day after her surgery and she was drug-free by April 1986. From February through April we took Mandy to the chiropractor three times a week. We began to see an enormous change in her health. In February when we decided to put Mandy's health totally in the chiropractor's care, she was very sick. She had a couple mild attacks the first few months, but when we would take her in for

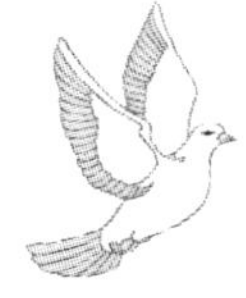

an adjustment, she had no side effects and she improved faster than she ever did before.

Chiropractic has most definitely changed our lives. Today, five years later, Mandy is an active and healthy child, thanks to Chiropractic care!

Mandy has taken three years of gymnastics, played softball for two years, and presently cheers for the Stockbridge Mighty-Mites. None of this would have been possible without her chiropractor and regular adjustments. In her last four and a half years, Mandy has not shown any signs of being asthmatic and has been an overall healthy child, requiring routine visits to her new pediatrician, the chiropractor.

Today, Robert, Mandy and I all see the chiropractor and have benefited enormously. We are all enjoying good health. In February 1986 Mandy's pediatrician told us he would not treat her again if we took her to a chiropractor. With regular Chiropractic care, she would no longer need him. We said, "Yes to Chiropractic!"

Without reservations we all recommend Chiropractic care FIRST for anyone suffering with any type of health problem.

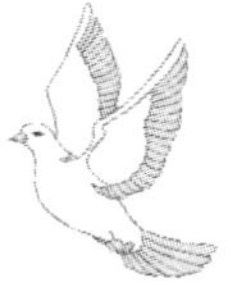

MENOPAUSE • *Lonna Mackie*

For more than two years it seemed as though I had been everywhere and to everyone trying to get assistance and advice on how I could feel better.

Because I am 50 years of age, I was informed that my problems were menopausal. I was told that there were certain measures that I could take to make this time in my life a little easier. These included hormone replacement therapy from my family physician, herbs from the naturopath, weekly visits to a massage therapist, daily walks, and workouts at the local health spa. I tried all of these with the exception of the hormone replacement therapy. They all worked to a certain extent, but I still did not feel like me.

I began going to the chiropractor in the first week of October 1994. We spoke of the type of treatment that he would be giving to me. I was skeptical. I even had the nerve to tell the chiropractor that I would try these treatments for two weeks only. That brief two week period was all that it took for me to begin to feel like the world had been lifted off my shoulders. I began sleeping through the night almost immediately. When I awoke in the morning, the customary stiffness in my shoulders and hips were no longer there.

I regained my interest in reading and in doing my crafts as my vision greatly improved in just a matter of weeks. The most wonderful

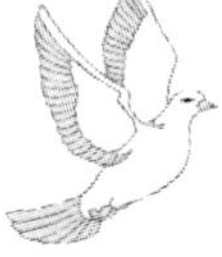

thing of all was that I began to notice that the stress of my job was not taking the toll on me that it had before. The tightness in my neck and upper back had begun to disappear. My job had not changed, I had. I also noticed that the people around me were happier and more fun to be around. They had not changed, I had.

I started to notice so many positive changes in my life that I began telling my family and friends about them. As I write this, I have not fully convinced all of them to begin treatments with the chiropractor, but I will not give up. I wish that everyone could feel as well as I do. I know for a fact that this feeling of well-being is a direct result of Chiropractic treatments. I have tried so many other types of treatments in my quest to feel better, but none of them have given me the results that I have enjoyed since I began Chiropractic care.

I am going to remain on this road to wellness for the rest of my life. I am so glad that the chiropractor has his clinic in North Bay. He has helped me to feel like me. Thank you.

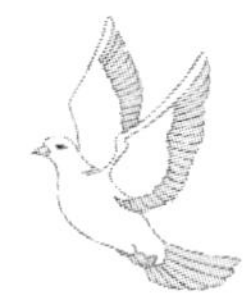

MENSTRUAL CRAMPS • *Melody Perry*

Hi, my name is Melody Perry. I am 14 years old. I have been visiting Dr. Yurick, a chiropractor, since October 1995. Before visiting Dr. Yurick, I always experienced excruciating cramps every month during my cycle. These cramps were so severe I was unable to attend school and important events.

I took medication to no avail, and the medical doctors told me that my cramps would stop after I had my first child. My mother took me to see the chiropractor. On my first visit to the chiropractor, he examined me and noticed my pelvis was tilted. After three visits to him for adjustments (which were not painful), when I had my period that month, I had no cramps.

I was completely pain free. I am very thankful to Chiropractic for curing my painful monthly cramps!

MY CHIROPRACTIC STORY

• *Derrick Moger*

Hi, my name is Derrick. I am eleven years old. I have asthma.

I don't like asthma, but I was born with it. So my mom and I decided to do something about it! I heard about the Firestone Clinic. My mom and I went to see what it was all about.

I had just had an asthma attack so I was on Prednisone. The Firestone Clinic said I couldn't be in the study, so my mom said: "What else can we do to help Derrick's asthma?" They recommended Cathy Wright and we found out where she was located.

We started going and having Chiropractic treatments, and it has helped me a lot. For example, I normally have a major asthma attack every three months, but after having Chiropractic treatments I have not had an asthma attack for five months. That is really, really good for me.

I am going to keep having Chiropractic treatments. I spend less time at the hospital and more time at home. That makes both me and my family very happy. Hopefully I can do a lot more things.

Chiropractic treatments really help my headaches, too. Once I had a major headache for about two days. I went to see Cathy. About five minutes after the treatment, my headache was just about gone. I think that is excellent.

I also went to camp for four days right when

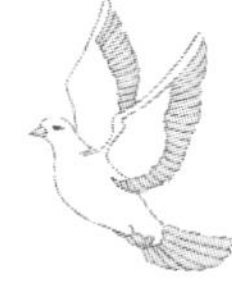

the tree pollen was at it's worst, and they had also cut the grass. Tree pollen and grass are two of my worst allergies. My mom and I were expecting me to come home and be sick for about a week, but I wasn't sick. I would go back to camp any day! Thanks to Chiropractic!

NO VOICE • *Chris Manceau*

No Voice! No longer could I enjoy doing what I was doing. I taught martial arts and was a bingo caller. The date: September 1990. My voice had begun to lose strength and continuity. After visiting with my family physician, he could not find anything wrong with me. Next was a referral to an ENT (ear, nose and throat) specialist. He, in turn, said everything was healthy. Perhaps a tonsillectomy might cure the problem. All this news came after 23 months of speech therapy. None of the treatments from these specialists had any effect.

The next step was to visit Toronto specialists and Sudbury neurologists in a continuous stream of appointments.

After months of not being able to communicate unless I whispered or spoke in spurts of three to four words, I changed family doctors. He referred me to my new chiropractor.

Now, after three adjustments, I can speak. Miracles happen.

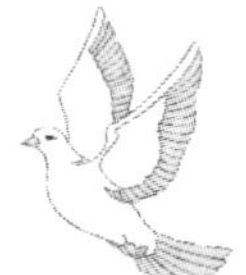

NO VOICE • *Margaret Moss*

For a period of two months I couldn't speak above a whisper. You can imagine how I coped working as a salesperson. The medical doctor I went to even put me in the hospital to do a biopsy to rule out cancer. Along with this, I had headaches over my eyes and neck stiffness. My biopsy report came back negative. I was grateful. The doctor told me that my loss of voice was caused by a pinched nerve in my neck. He gave me pills to take and I wondered how taking pills would correct a pinched nerve. The answer was it didn't. The pain continued, and I still had no voice.

While talking to a friend who once suffered from a pinched nerve, I was told to see the chiropractor who had helped her. The doctor took two X-rays of my neck and showed me where he felt the nerve was being pinched. In two days my voice started getting stronger, and in two weeks my voice was real strong.

I can not speak highly enough of Chiropractic. I would urge all people who have pinched nerves to go see a chiropractor.

I asked my doctor why the medical doctor didn't send me to a chiropractor when he knew I had a pinched nerve. He said for the same reason a Ford dealer doesn't recommend buying a Chevy … kind of makes sense.

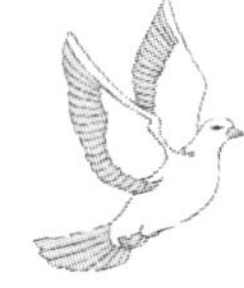

OUR MIRACLE SON • *Marie-Claire Groulx*

Children are born every minute of every day. They are created and given to parents as gifts. It is up to us to choose how we will raise these little people regardless of the difficulties life may throw at us.

On the day we moved into our new home, my family physician confirmed that I was pregnant. We were very happy. The pregnancy progressed and the nausea subsided, but in my tummy, along with my baby, was another growth, something growing bigger and faster than the baby. Around four months of pregnancy, I was referred to an obstetrician. I had to wait a few days for an appointment. During one of these nights I experienced intense abdominal pain. People had been praying for me. When I saw the doctor the following day, the growth had disappeared mysteriously.

Time went on and I soon became huge. At seven months contractions started, three minutes apart, then one minute apart. I went to the hospital frightened that I might lose the baby. I was put on an alcohol drip and then was injected with lung stimulating hormones for my baby. After five days of bed rest, I went home.

At eight months I was readmitted with a dangerously low estral level – below the life-sustaining level. We pulled through this and went home after six days of total bed rest.

Finally, three days after my due date, I began labor. My water broke, and I had strong

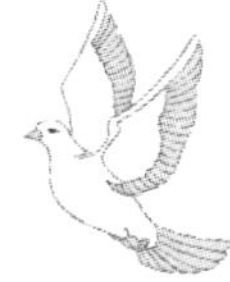

contractions that began near midnight. We went to the hospital, and contractions continued, one minute apart, from 12 a.m. till noon, then 30 seconds apart. They decided to section me. I was in shock, my baby was in a breach position in fetal distress. I was four centimeters dilated, tired and scared. After an epidural I was wheeled into the O.R. and given a quick section while I was awake. Our beautiful, curly-haired, pink son was born at 8:20 p.m., perfect and healthy. In my womb they found a large scar, a remnant of whatever had been growing there: a mystery, a miracle. Francois came home after six days. He had been quite jaundiced but nursed well.

Time went on, and he gained weight quickly. He was a real fussy baby and any change would upset him.

He began having his teeth at three months and was very ill with every tooth. At six months he was admitted to the hospital with a diaper full of bloody mush. He was so ill. Every doctor in town it seemed had seen him and couldn't understand what was wrong. The next day he cut three teeth at once and we all felt better. The fever went down, and he began to drink again.

His health was up and down; he was often sick. Our family doctor was concerned with his slow growth pattern, low weight, his many colds, his persistent earaches, infections, etc. We were frequent visitors to the doctor's office, but had no other options offered to us. We did the best

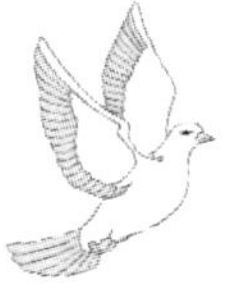

we knew how. Francois's hearing was sometimes less than 40% in his early years in school. He was treated by an ear, nose, throat specialist for several years. He had tubes in his ears five times and a tonsillectomy after several cases of pneumonia.

At age six, after several bouts of infection, he had a circumcision. Post-op infection meant a long stay in hospital. At age seven he spent nearly five months in total in hospital for several bouts of asthma, pneumonia, lung collapses, etc. From this point on, he was considered a chronic asthmatic. We went to Ottawa for a visit to a special clinic for lung disorders. He was treated with a variety of medications, with various effects.

From age seven to fifteen Francois was a frequent visitor to pediatrics at St. Joseph's Hospital. On average he had four or five cases of pneumonia a year and three or four lung collapses. Beside everything else, he had chicken pox, influenza and infections. He was taking seven to twelve different kinds of medications a day, up to six times a day. Physiotherapy was part of our home routine. Life was lived one day at a time for those eight years. Our whole family life revolved around health and trying to achieve it.

Our pediatrician was wonderful support to us; nonetheless, I was always open to new ways of improving my family's health. During the spring of 1994, while visiting a naturopathic doctor for myself, I received suggestions in

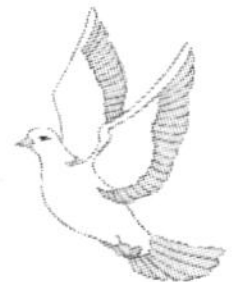

caring for asthmatics: changes in diet. Francois visited the naturopath and was prescribed a bottle of homeopathic preparation to stimulate metabolism in his digestive system.

After having seen many doctors in North Bay and Ottawa for a recurring neurological disorder, I still had a poor quality of life. I finally decided to try a chiropractor in addition to the naturopath. I chose Dr. Thomas Preston. Within a few visits I noticed a remarkable improvement in my energy level as well as my co-ordination. I thought immediately of Francois who had been diagnosed with scoliosis, and asked Dr. Preston if he would consider treating him. Treatment began within days.

After six months, no more medications, no colds, no more asthma. Wow! Life force surged through him to stimulate his immune system. One year nearly to the day after a double lung collapse, a subcutaneous pneumothorax in his first days of high school, Francois and I learned he officially had no more asthma. He had officially been given a ten percent chance, at best, of ever outgrowing this kind of asthma in his life. Chronic asthma challenges many children.

Now, his quality of life has improved. He is medication free. Even his dentist has seen an improvement in his oral health. Medications have side effects that linger in the system and can be annoying. No more.

In early December of this year, Francois woke up feeling very sick. With early cold

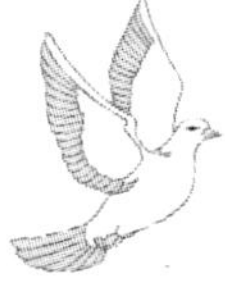

symptoms I was concerned that he might become very ill, as he had many, many times before. Off we went to our chiropractor's office for an adjustment. He seemed to stabilize, then his condition deteriorated within twelve hours. He woke up on Saturday morning with a partial lung collapse. I telephoned Dr. Preston at home, and within the hour Francois was being adjusted. We went home thankful. We exercised. We walked while doing deep breathing. We drank a lot of water. After six hours, Francois was breathing normally. His lung had reinflated. He was tiring easily, but he was able to rest comfortably. What a miracle!

We are still aiming for physical growth. To have suffered as he has and be where he is now is truly a miracle. Our entire family receives Chiropractic care from Dr. Preston. He truly is a very special caring man who inspires wellness in all his patients.

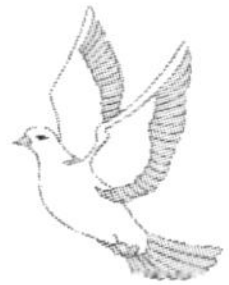

PARALYSIS • *Elana Brown, D.C.*

About 50 years ago my father was in engineering in college, Michigan Tech, studying for a degree in mechanical engineering. During that time, he was in a major car accident and became paralyzed from the waist up. Medical doctors said that surgery was his only choice and that this could be done for about $400. That kind of money was not available to him at that time.

One of his football team mates suggested he try Chiropractic and try his chiropractor. My father weighed over 210 pounds in those days. He could not move the upper parts of his body: his shoulders didn't move, he couldn't lift his arms and he couldn't turn his neck. The chiropractor was an old, small man who gave a standard adjustment. My father said it was the most painful adjustment of his life. After the adjustment he was able to move all of his upper body.

He continued under Chiropractic care for several visits to make sure that his spinal problem was corrected. He loved Chiropractic. From then on, as he graduated from school and worked in sales at a large engineering supply house, he constantly told people about Chiropractic. This helped people from problems ranging from headaches, sinusitis and bronchitis to paralysis problems. He sent hundreds of people to chiropractors.

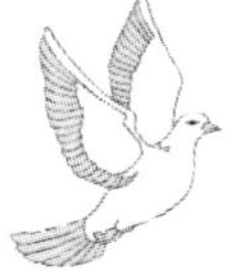

He found a chiropractor when he moved back to Brooklyn, New York. I know that they became good friends in time.

Lou knew how much my father was talking about Chiropractic so he wrote a letter to B. J. Palmer, the son of the founder of Chiropractic. Palmer sent my father a card which said:

"Please give the bearer of this card, ***Bernard Brown***, adjustments, and if you want to be paid I will pay – because this person has been doing a great amount of good for Chiropractic."

My father went into the army air corps as an engineering officer and married my mother. He made sure she took adjustments, and as they had children, they were also under Chiropractic care.

In 1954 my father went back to night school to become a chiropractor. He had his engineering job by day, supported his wife and three children and went to school at night. It was no surprise to us that by the time he graduated from school he changed careers—from engineering to Chiropractic.

This is written by his youngest daughter. I have been adjusted since birth and almost never have been given medication. I have lived a Chiropractic lifestyle. I am also a chiropractor.

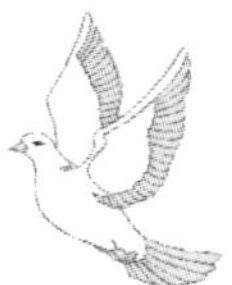

POLIO • *Mrs. Linda McInnis*

Dear Readers,

I'm a forty-four-year-old woman who was born and inflicted during the Polio Epidemic. For years I have lived with pain and discomfort and have had many surgeries. I have suffered with migraine headaches, swelling of joints in my arms and legs, spasms and weakness, severe back pain, sinus problems, and chest pain.

The doctors have told me that because of polio this was to be expected. They sent me to physiotherapy and to a psychologist. Next they would give me medication. Then the pain would come back.

I have seen many doctors in my life, as I move often because of my husband's job. This time I found a doctor who really listened and understood how I felt. He asked me to consider Chiropractic treatment. I was very skeptical.

My preliminary examination was on October 6, 1994. The doctor went over my records and X-rays. He explained what the treatment involved and how it worked. He explained that there are twenty-four vertebrae in your spine and that most of mine were subluxated. The nerves were being interfered with and damaged. He then explained that every nerve had a purpose and that each one interfered with would cause different symptoms. This meant we had a lot of work ahead of us to repair the damage.

I realize that I'm far from being completely

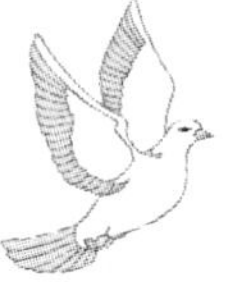

healthy, but it is very nice to live without so much pain. Since October, I've had only one minor headache, and the swelling has gone down in my hands and legs. I now can sleep at night, and I have more energy to do the things I enjoy. I have not had a cold or the flu since I began treatment. For me this is great, as I usually have bronchitis or pneumonia at least once or twice a year.

As for my neck and shoulders, I now have mobility up to 80%. Before I would have to turn my whole body to see things beside me. Once a year I would have cortisone shots in both shoulders just to keep them mobile. For me, my chiropractors, along with their staff, have changed my life. I am very thankful to them for their support and friendship. The cheerful way they greet you at the door every morning makes you feel very special and important.

Thank you Chiropractic!

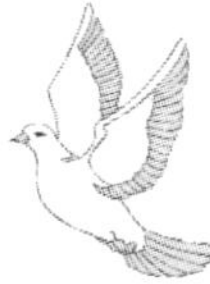

REFLUX DISEASE • *Tom McCann*

In 1960 I had an automobile accident from which I escaped with nothing broken except a couple of teeth. Subsequent to that accident, I suffered for 30 years with a choking condition which occurred during eating. I did not connect the choking with the accident.

In the early years, the problem was diagnosed as esophagitis. The quantity or quality of the food eaten seemed to have nothing to do with the problem. Nor did the speed with which food was consumed have any bearing upon the difficulty. In those days, I would suffer an attack every few months. For a number of years, I had no attacks.

A few years ago, the attacks started again. This time the condition was diagnosed by two medical doctors as Reflux Disease brought on by massive heart burn. Since I had never had heart burn (I believe that it is painful), the diagnosis seemed unrealistic. The doctor prescribed a special diet, supplemented with Axid and Prepulsid. The Axid was supposed to reduce the amount of stomach acid produced after eating. The Prepulsid was supposed to strengthen the sphincter at the bottom of the esophagus.

The frequency of the attacks or episodes increased. The medication was working. The sphincter was so strong that it would shut down at the hint of food. I believe that I was having esophageal muscle spasms, where the muscles did not work in sequence (as in peristalsis), but

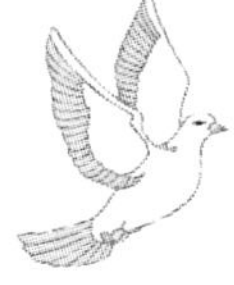

tightened up all at once. I could not eat.

Then the duration of the episodes went beyond four or five hours; I started going to the hospital each time. In the hospital they tried a combination of valium, morphine, glucagon, nitro glycerin and the stuff they give for sea sickness. None of it worked more than once. The Prepulsid had made the muscles too strong. The only thing that worked was toughing it out and standing over a sink for 10 to 11 hours. Remember, all this time I was unable to swallow anything, including my own saliva or water. Water brought on a really violent wretching, so I stopped that as well.

During a one-week vacation trip to New Brunswick, the episodes struck every day or so. My family regarded me as some sort of time bomb that had to jump up and leave restaurants at a moment's notice.

Upon returning from the East coast, at the end of August, 1995, I went immediately to my doctor. He suggested that they could run the tests again. From the doctor's office, I went straight to a naturopathic practitioner who in turn sent me straight to a Chiropractor. Both of those people had seen the condition or similar conditions previously, and it had been treatable.

I am happy to report that under Chiropractic care, and a change in diet, I am now a healed man.

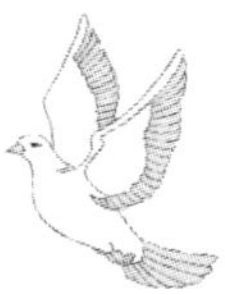

RHEUMATOID ARTHRITIS

• *Agnes B. Jourdin*

On July 4, 1960, I watched my granddaughter Patti playing in a sand box. As she moved about, it became obvious that something was wrong with her right knee. The thought flashed through my mind this was the way I remembered the crippling onset of arthritis that I experienced in my youth. A sickening feeling of despair and hopelessness surged through me.

On Monday I called my physician and made an appointment for Patti. After a thorough examination he recommended further tests be made at the Pediatric Clinic of New York Hospital. On July 22 she was admitted to the clinic and a nightmare: tests and examinations by X-ray, blood studies and numerous needles began. At first our visits were once a week, then later once a month. After each of these sessions Patti came home more fearful and more exhausted. The culmination of the examinations ruled out everything except the condition was either tuberculosis of the bone or rheumatoid arthritis.

Patti was then referred to the Arthritis Clinic of the Hospital for Special Surgery. After a conference between the doctors of both hospitals, the conclusion was reached that a positive diagnosis of rheumatoid arthritis could not be made until one or more joints became infected. In this event, it was decided, a series of gold salt injections would be administered.

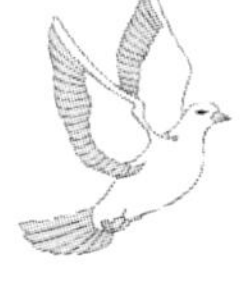

A complete leg brace from hip to foot was made for Patti's leg. The orthopedic clinic said she must wear this when actively engaged in play. Hot packs on the knee were to be applied three times a day for a half hour at a time.

In January 1961 the left knee began to swell. I knew this confirmed the diagnosis of rheumatoid arthritis. From my own experience I knew that meant painful weekly gold salt injections and blood tests every month or six weeks. The futility of such treatment was evident in my own case, and we desperately sought another approach. Chiropractic was suggested to us, and on February 20, 1961, both Patti and I entered the office of Dr. Robert Oerzen for Chiropractic care.

One of the first things our chiropractor suggested after Patti had her first adjustment, was complete freedom to play without the brace. To be able to leave her wheel chair and play with other children, instead of watching them, seemed too good to be true! It became true! Patti was able to play, and her legs got better steadily. Her swollen little knees shrunk back to normal. Small wonder she adores her "Dr. Bob."

Patti is now six and a half years of age. On September 13 of this year she was required to have a medical examination for school. When her mother told the doctor that she had rheumatoid arthritis, he checked her thoroughly. His remark was, "Whoever your doctor was he did a remarkable job here. I find no trace of arthritis."

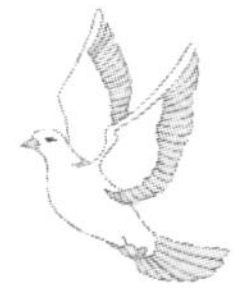

When he was told that it was Chiropractic treatment that corrected Patti's condition, he examined her again. Finally he replied, "I hate to admit it, but it's true, there is no trace of arthritis now."

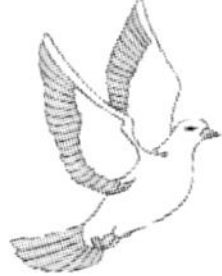

RHEUMATOID ARTHRITIS

• *Elizabeth Jones*

Dear Dr. Andy,

I am writing you this letter to thank you. Without your care and wonderful treatments my life would not be as fulfilling as it is. When I first came to your office, my life and daily activities were limited to being confined to my home and only short trips to the grocery store.

I suffered from extreme arthritis in my hands, leaving me almost unable to even lift a milk carton to fill my grandchildren's glasses. I also had severe pain and stiffness in every joint in my body. My medical doctor, who I had been going to for years, was only able to keep subscribing different pain killers and anti-inflammatory drugs, which gave me only temporary relief. The pain was so bad at night, I was unable to get more than two hours of sleep at a time.

My son convinced me to try Chiropractic. I was at my wits' end and was willing to try anything. After my first several adjustments, I was unsure that it was going to help since I was so sore after each one. But I stuck with it, and I can't believe the difference.

Dr. Andy, I want to thank you for giving me back what I had thought I could never have again. Now I am able to watch my grandchildren all day, walk around the mall without pain, and cook and clean like I had years ago. I only wish I knew Dr. Andy 20 years ago. Thanks again!

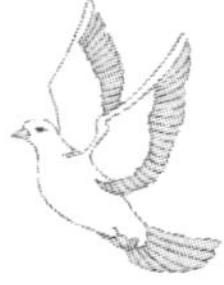

SCOLIOSIS • *Allison Beller-Bernsten*

I was diagnosed with scoliosis. I wore a Milwaukee brace for four years. I had pain in my entire back, headaches, numbness of hands and feet, and chest pains.

As a child I was under the care of an orthopedic clinic. Before Chiropractic I had seen in internist who could not help with the chest pains or headaches.

A friend had been helped a great deal through Chiropractic care after injuring his spine in a car accident. He suggested that I make an appointment with the chiropractor.

The chiropractor found that I had subluxations of the entire spine, rotations of the spinal vertebrae and calcium spurs. This doctor also found that my neck had been injured due to an accident years before. This was causing the headaches.

Since I started receiving Chiropractic treatments, I no longer have the severe pain. My energy level is higher than ever before, and my general health is great. *I am no longer moody or depressed.*

It is an important part of good health. This is not all I have received from my chiropractor. He also gives great advice on nutrition and exercise, and supports and inspires his patients toward having a healthy, active life.

Chiropractic is for everyone.

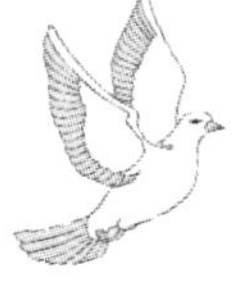

SCOLIOSIS • *Duncan Stewart's Story*

I had a scoliosis operation in 1979. A Harrinton Rod was placed in my back. I was then put into a body cast for nine months. During this time (I was only 14 years old) I thought when the cast was removed I would feel fine, be healthy and go on with my life. However, that was just the beginning of my troubles. Medically maybe my spine was corrected, but I was still a mess.

I was not standing straight, headaches were frequent, neck pain and shoulder discomfort were always present. I lived the most important part of my growing adolescent years in pain, discomfort and not feeling healthy. Sleeping was a problem. Getting comfortable in a position to sleep was a big project, rather than being able to hit the bed and go to sleep.

Not knowing much about Chiropractic care and having a foreign object placed in my back, I didn't know what to do with myself. Finally in 1987 my brother recommended a chiropractor. I very nervously but willingly went to meet you and discuss my life with you.

The first step was to have a full examination including X-rays and to evaluate my problems. The chiropractor went step by step with each procedure, fully explaining everything that was done. The professionalism and understanding of my fears of somebody touching and adjusting my spine meant a lot to me. I already had undergone major surgery and still was in discomfort.

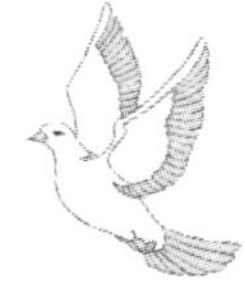

Can something else actually be done to help me? This is what I used to wonder.

Well, doctor, after all these years, YOU, yes YOU! have answered all those questions. You have helped me to overcome any fears that I had about Chiropractic care. You have helped me to know and feel what it means to be healthy. Through your constant caring and proper Chiropractic attention, I now am functioning like a normal, healthy human being and IT FEELS GREAT!

I wouldn't want anyone to have to suffer as I did. Had I known and understood Chiropractic care sooner, maybe it would have been the answer in place of surgery.

SEIZURES • *Juana Rivera*

I decided to give Chiropractic a try after talking to a friend for the sake of my eight-year-old son Michael. Michael has suffered from seizures, three or four per week for six years! As a result, his vocal chords were damaged, and he completely lost his speech. In addition Michael couldn't walk, stand or even hold up his head.

Thank God, after four months of Chiropractic with Dr. Roses, Michael has had only three seizures. Now he is up and around. He is able to walk freely. He's also trying to speak by making babbling sounds. He seems to be happy. His progress is already a miracle!

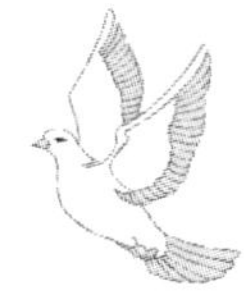

SPINA BIFIDA • *Duncan Stewart*

I was born on July 7, 1960, with Spina Bifida Occulta and scoliosis. I was also born with a clubbed foot. Life as a child was filled with the usual examinations with an orthopedic surgeon and eventually I was scheduled for a spinal fusion when I was ten years old. The fusion was at the fourth and fifth lumbar vertebra. This fusion prevented my scoliosis from continuing it's course. The doctor stated that without the surgery I was probably going to end up severing my spinal cord.

As a ten-year-old boy it is very difficult to explain to an adult as well as a surgeon that I felt the surgery was not necessary. Having said that, I went on with life and was going along fine until a car accident on August 19, 1988. My car was rear-ended, and over a short period of time my back started to give me problems.

I had pain radiating down my legs, particularly on the left side. My buttocks were sore. I had no energy. I was really concerned about my walking, as I was having trouble going up and down stairs. I needed to hold onto the railing to support myself. I was fearful of ending up in a wheelchair. I couldn't do any business at all.

I went to my doctor and he recommended muscle relaxants, pain killers and physiotherapy. The muscle relaxants didn't work. The pain killers made me want to sleep. The physiotherapy didn't work either.

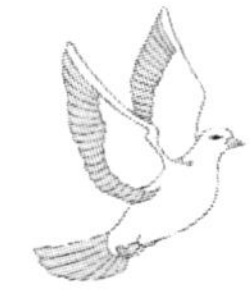

My doctor then sent me to an orthopedic surgeon. The orthopedic surgeon preferred to send me to a neurologist. The end result of the two meetings I had with him was once again surgery. His answer to my constant pain was to burn the nerves in my spine that were causing the discomfort.

If that was what it was going to take, I could handle it. I was given a fifty-fifty chance of the surgery working and those weren't the odds that I was looking for, so I called a friend in California who is a chiropractor. I filled him in on the problem I was having ,and he told me to go to a chiropractor in Toronto. I told him of my apprehension with regard to any doctor at this point, and he assured me that it would not hurt me more than I was already feeling. At that point I took his advice and was waiting for him to call me back with a couple of phone numbers of chiropractors in my area. He phoned and told me to get on a plane and get to his clinic in Santa Rosa, California.

I was with him for one month, and I will say that the change in my health as well as appearance was amazing. Naturally, nothing happens over night. When I got back to Toronto, I phoned a customer of mine and inquired about her chiropractor. She recommended Dr. Brett in Oakville, Ontario.

I phoned his office and made an appointment to see him. From the first moment I met Brett, I knew that I had found my answer to my back problems. Today, five years later I have never felt so well.

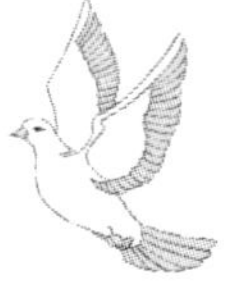

I have sent my two brothers to chiropractors since I started, and they can't stop talking about the positive results. They, as well as myself, are walking billboards of Chiropractic. We talk to anybody that will listen about the positive effects.

Today, after many needed adjustments, I have seen many physical changes with my body. My gait has improved. My energy level is higher than ever. I have more mobility. I now run up a set of stairs, two steps at a time.

If I can change the public's attitude about Chiropractic, it will be worth it. I can tell you that I have changed many people's attitudes since I started with Chiropractic. All that people have to do is look at me now and review pictures of my youth through to my accident in 1988.

I have been accepted to Life College in Marietta, Georgia to study Chiropractic. To change one's career at my age says something about my feelings toward the art and science of Chiropractic. I invite anyone with a problem with their back to see a Doctor of Chiropractic before taking the last resort of surgery.

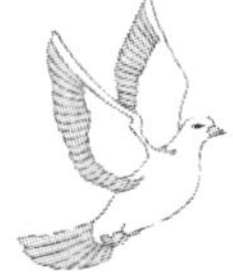

STILL SEARCHING FOR HEALTH

• *Rose-Alda Villetier*

I am 86 years old, and last spring I was crippled with a constant pain in my legs and my back. I couldn't walk without using a cane and was awake most of the night. My daughter encouraged me to see a chiropractor because I wasn't getting any better with the medication prescribed by my family doctor.

Even if I was not convinced, I decided to visit Doctor Tom. At the beginning of the treatments I was still in pain and very discouraged! But eventually and gradually after eight or nine weeks of treatments, the pain has completely disappeared.

Thanks to Doctor Tom, who came to my rescue, I feel like a very well person and enjoy living a healthy life again.

Thank God I'm ALIVE !

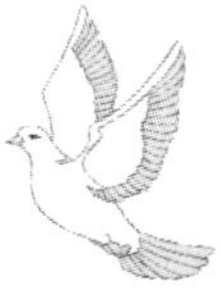

STOMACH PROBLEMS • *Scott Hanley*

Can Chiropractic Care Help Me?

At first I believed it couldn't. Since I was in fifth grade, I have had stomach trouble: tightness of my stomach and frequent diarrhea.

I am now in the eleventh grade. For those six years I have tried different medicines and doctors to try to solve my stomach troubles. All those attempts were unsuccessful.

I then went to the chiropractors with little hope. I did not think that they could solve stomach problems. They explained to me what was wrong and how they were going to fix it.

At first it got worse, but in a month's time I was feeling totally better.

Thanks to the chiropractors, my life-long problem was solved.

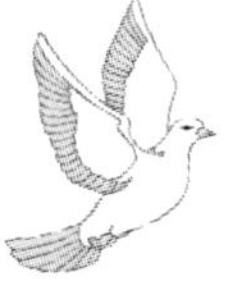

STOMACH TROUBLE • *J. F. Porter*

It gives me great pleasure to give this testimonial of what Chiropractic and the chiropractor have done for my health. During most of my life I have had stomach trouble, but for the past two years my stomach trouble has been very bad. It had gotten so bad that eating any food would cause severe pain and upset. In two-years' time six doctors treated me for stomach trouble and ulcers, but nothing seemed to help. You can imagine how I felt to have to work hard as a mechanic and not be able to amount to much of anything.

One day a friend of mine was telling me about going to the chiropractor and about the results. I decided to try for myself, as nothing else had helped me. The chiropractor took X-rays and checked me over. He showed me the cause of my trouble and started Chiropractic treatments. In three weeks the problems started leaving, and I was able to eat. By the end of two months, all of my stomach pain left, and I was eating anything that I wanted.

It is now 18 months since the chiropractor first worked on me, and I am still well. My weight has picked up from 145 to 175 lb. Chiropractic has helped me like nothing else could. I sure do urge other sick people to try it. I like the way it gets at the cause of the problem.

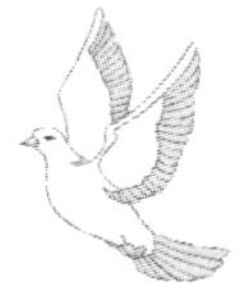

THE DEMANDS OF A BROADWAY BEAUTY • *Marla Trump*

When the demands of a Broadway career took their physical toll on me, I sought the expertise of Dr. Michael C. Smatt in New York City. In the show there are 50 steps that we dance up and down, and I do cartwheels, splits and tap dancing in the choreography. I felt a lot of stress in my hips, knees and back. I found the stress on my body was incredible.

Then I heard about Dr. Smatt, and he taught me the basic philosophy of Chiropractic. It made more and more sense as time went on. I had very good results with Chiropractic and by the time I was doing two shows a day, I found the adjustments to be energizing.

Faced with long hours and grueling performance regimes, performers have to muster incredible stamina. When the day starts you have to be aware of your body, and you have to be in tune with it. You have to breathe and stretch properly, and you have to take time to stop, to be quiet and feel the muscles stretch. Because I hadn't stretched the muscles, I developed bad hamstring pulls and sciatica, but Dr. Smatt helped me get over it.

While I was pregnant with my daughter Tiffany, I got regular Chiropractic adjustments to give the baby every chance to be healthy. Since then, I have made Chiropractic care a family priority. My daughter Tiffany gets adjusted once a month, and I have referred many friends

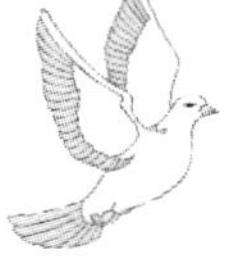

to Dr. Smatt.

Dr. Smatt utilizes diversified upper cervical techniques to provide care for his patients who are often musicians and dancers. "Most of the performers that come to me need to relieve stress in the nervous system. Restoring optimal function of the nervous system lets them give a better performance."

In preparation for a tour or stage performance, my schedule of care increases. I see my chiropractor more frequently because of the physical trauma of the performances. A performer has to develop mental toughness, and I believe in positive thinking to clear the obstacles. I believe the mental aspect has a much more powerful influence than we know. I believe in meditation and I understand the philosophy of the power within us to heal ourselves.

A regular exercise schedule helps alleviate stress. Despite having to deal with the press about my private life, which is often more public than I would sometimes like, I am determined to find outlets for my numerous talents.

I would love to learn more about health, fitness and to give more back to the people and the industry who have given to me. My goal is to educate myself and others, spreading the message about physical fitness and well-being to the world. That is where my focus is. Reaching physical, mental and spiritual fitness is a journey; you just don't learn it overnight.

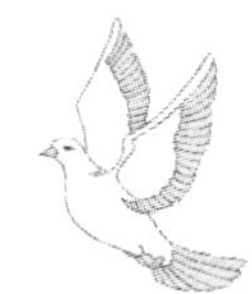

TRIGEMINAL NERVE DISEASE

• *Gloria Steinem's Story*

Recognized for her crucial and significant work for women's rights, Gloria Steinem was listed in the World Almanac's "25 Most Influential Women in America" and in 1993 she was inducted into the National Women's Hall of Fame. Acknowledged also for her scholarly work, Gloria Steinem was awarded the first Doctorate of Human Justice, awarded by Simmons College. She received many awards for civil liberties, as well as the Liberty Award of the the Lambda Legal Defense and Education Fund and the Ceres Medal from the United Nations.

One would not expect her to be a spokesperson for alternative health care. In most intellectual and political circles, she is regarded for her feminist philosophy, rather than her healing viewpoints.

Gloria Steinem sees a parallel, "as women historically were the healers in many cultures. This is the reason that they were burned at the stake as witches, because they were healers. So certainly the two are very much connected."

"My grandmother had always gone to a chiropractor and believed in Chiropractic much more than in conventional medicine," she emphasizes. Like so many people who depend on traditional medicine and wait to seek out alternative care until they've reached a point of desperation, she found something that works in combining Chiropractic with nutrition.

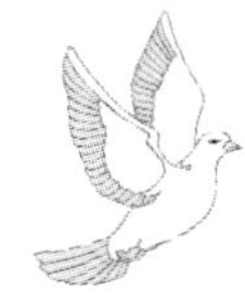

As her parents did not share the same view, she was only tangibly aware of the care.

"From the time I was in high school, I had back problems, because I had one extra lumbar vertebrae, which meant that my back was just a tiny bit lopsided, perhaps," she recalls. "I had back spasms once a year or so, and that solved itself over time. But I continued to have some neck, shoulder and back stress partly because of sitting at my computer all day, I suppose."

In 1995 Steinem was forced to curtail her writing activities when she contracted a rare nerve disease, trigeminal neuralgia, and found that the mundane activities in her life became a menace. She was forced to cancel her national tour to promote her new book, "Moving Beyond Words," because of the excruciating pain in her jaw and face. Eating and speaking became unbearable for her.

"It almost always begins as a terrific, traumatic tooth pain. You bite down and you have to think this is the worst tooth pain in the world," she says. "So what usually happens is that poor people have their teeth out and rich people have root canals, and then discover that the pain continues anyway, which is what happened to me. I had one unnecessary root canal."

Steinem's dentist then sent her to a neurologist, who finally diagnosed the problem as trigeminal neuralgia and prescribed medication that is used for epileptic seizures.

"That worked for about a day, but you had to keep taking more of it," recalls Steinem,

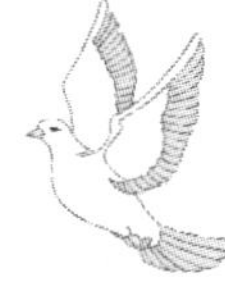

adding that the side effects were awful. "It makes you feel fuzzy and headachy, so I just stopped taking it and tried to deal with it in other ways."

There were other options presented to her that were even less desirable. "The most frequent surgical way of dealing with this is to deaden the nerves in the cheek so that you don't feel the pain," she says.

The electric needle injections would leave a permanently diminished feeling in the cheek. Unfortunately, even with this treatment the pain usually comes back. The second and more recent surgical method was even more extreme … brain surgery. After drilling a hole at the back of the brain, the surgeon reaches in to the trigeminal nerve in the forehead, separates it from the vein that is pressing on it, and wraps the nerve in Teflon.

"I was not going to do that unless there was no other alternative," Gloria emphasized. Fortunately there was another approach. She was referred to a Manhattan chiropractor, Dr. Michael Smatt, who began providing care for her in February of 1995.

When Steinem came in for her first visit, Smatt suggested that she discontinue using the medication Tegretol that had been prescribed to her so that her body could function at optimum.

He took upper cervical X-rays and discovered that her atlas and axis subluxations were causing pressure on the brain stem. In addition Dr. Smatt utilized an innovative procedure, Contact Reflex Analysis (CRA) which is a

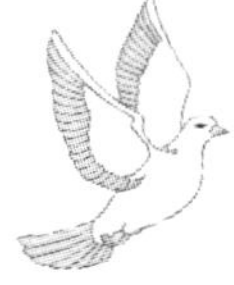

method of evaluating the combination of structural, physical and nutritional needs within the body. "Any deficiency in any of the areas could cause or contribute to various acute or chronic health care problems," Smatt explains.

Pointing out that CRA is not a method of diagnosis, Smatt describes the procedure as a means by which health care professionals can use the body reflexes to determine the root causes of the health problem. This procedure has been taught in continuing education seminars across the US for more than thirty years.

During the analysis of Steinem, Dr. Smatt found that her parotid, or chemical poisoning reflex was weak, which is common when the immune system is not functioning well.

"When functioning normally, the parotid hormones stimulate the production of saliva, which neutralizes the toxins and digests the bacteria and chemicals before they reach the digestive system," Smatt explains, adding that these hormones are also important to the health of teeth and gums.

In addressing his findings, Dr. Smatt gave Steinem atlas and axis-specific adjustments three times a week and recommended that she take specific nutritional supplements for approximately twelve weeks.

Now experiencing total relief from the disorder, she is thankful for the results and states, "It took three months to be able to function and four months for it to go away completely, but I did not have to undergo surgery!"

In assessing Chiropractic, Steinem praises

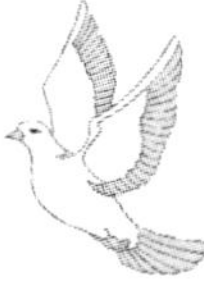

the big picture. "Certainly in other health care approaches, you tend to focus on the part that is malfunctioning rather than on the whole body," she points out.

Gloria Steinem believes that society's indoctrination to the traditional medical paradigm as well as lack of individual responsibility for health care are the causes of a health situation that is desperate. Health care should address the problems for a holistic viewpoint, encompassing nutrition and Chiropractic.

"It will help all of us, men and women, to focus on espousing alternative health care approaches that concentrate on a life cycle model, from pediatrics to geriatrics. We must look at the whole body and increase our trust of our own bodies," Steinem says.

Only a little while ago, Gloria Steinem had no control over talking, eating or traveling. With Chiropractic care, this mentor to millions, both men and women alike, was able to move beyond the pain and once more be an international figure of her time.

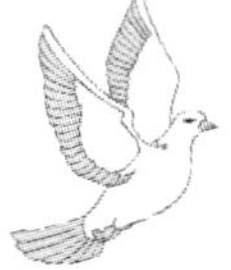

THE JOURNEY CONTINUES

• *Hollis Griffith*

I have had steady pain throughout my body for as long as I can remember. Sometimes it was very severe. The pain was mostly located in my shoulders, legs, chest, arms, back and even my feet.

I was seeing an internist who put me on medication but also led me to my decision to see Dr. Sirlin. I had never been to a chiropractor and was very hesitant until I spoke to my daughter about Dr. Sirlin.

After seeing this chiropractor, I understood why my daughter recommended him so highly. The service was great and everyone at the office was so cheerful. He made many recommendations which have had good results so far. My wife noticed the improvement in me and decided to become a patient due to the fact that she also had pain throughout her body. Since then, she has been gardening, which is something she hasn't done for years.

I would recommend to anyone who is sick or suffering pain to see a chiropractor. Since seeing Dr. Sirlin I have achieved better health.

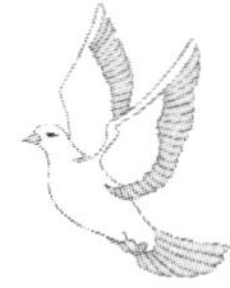

WRY NECK SYNDROME • *Harry Fogarty*

Dear Doctor,

I was relieved of the pain immediately and one of the fringe benefits I got was when crossing the street, I was able to walk instead of shuffling like an old man. One day I was sitting in the chair in the back yard, and all of a sudden I had a feeling: I was just feeling good!

The other night I walked around a bazaar for two hours without getting tired or dragging my feet or anything else. I wasn't looking for all this health. All I was looking for was a doctor who could get rid of the pain in my shoulder. I went in for the pain in my shoulder, and I shuffled. Everyone called me Tim Conway. Instead of shuffling like that, I can actually walk full steps. I'm really amazed at it myself.

I guess I could have always done it, but the strength just wasn't there. Something was wrong with my body that I wasn't connected to it right. The chiropractor turns the energy on, just like watering your garden. When I first came here, I was a skeptic, a real skeptic. I figured I'll let this quack take a whack at it. Now, I'm really so glad I did it. I can't express how much it means to me.

I guess "Thank God" for chiropractors, otherwise I'd be shuffling till I died.

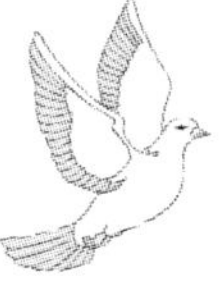

WRY NECK SYNDROME • *Eileen Lutz*

I clearly remember the first time I experienced the painful spasm in my neck and shoulder. I was 18 years old, and the pain was so intense that I went immediately to my family doctor for treatment. At that time, he speculated that I had "caught a draft" from an open car window. He sent me home with instructions to rest with a heating pad on my back until the stiffness subsided. I tried the treatment, and eventually my shoulder got better.

Unfortunately, no matter how careful I was, the pain and stiffness would resurface every now and then without warning. Throughout college and the various jobs I've had over the years, I would invariably end up in some simple situation that would result in experiencing pain, migraine headache and "frozen shoulder." The more sophisticated internists X-rayed my cervical spine and diagnosed "wry neck syndrome" and advised me to rest at home until the stiffness subsided.

By the time I reached 30, I couldn't remember a day when I had not felt pain in my shoulder. I would lose several days of work each month. The new, young internist advised me that torticollis continues to worsen with age and that I would probably have to live with the pain and bad posture the rest of my life. His best advice was not to lift anything heavier than an empty plate. To help me hold my head relatively erect during the worst of it, he had me fitted for

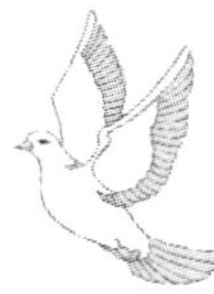

a cervical collar.

During the third bout of serious pain in less than four weeks, I received a call from my boss who carried on almost endlessly about Chiropractic. He had gone to a chiropractor himself. This wasn't just any chiropractor, he was the best one around. I should call and make an appointment right away. Of course, when your boss is paying you for staying home and he calls you especially to recommend a particular doctor to help you get back on your feet, you have to do the right thing and make the call. I did.

Andrew was the first and only doctor to take me, my posture and my pain seriously. Because Andrew took the time to work with me as closely as he did, I felt there was a real possibility for recovery. I also knew I could trust him enough to literally lay my life in his hands.

It took a very long time and many visits with Andrew before the day came when, magically, I suddenly realized that I had been pain-free all day. That was the first of many days to follow, first sporadically, then frequently. Finally the pain became the exception rather than the rule.

After more than 10 years of constant pain, I am now able to move my head freely and painlessly. Those who dare to talk down about Chiropractic in my presence have met the wrath of its staunchest supporter. I am living proof that Chiropractic does work.

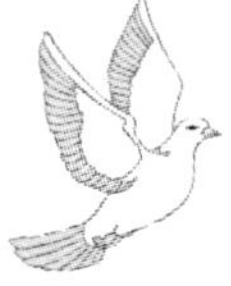

Part Three

Closing Thoughts

In reading these stories, we see that the life and light of the miracles of the body can transform our earthly nature. Children, adults and the elderly have had a second chance, a fresh start at being alive on our planet.

The Life and Times of the modern day genius, B.J. Palmer, will some day be told more fully. His story, the triumphs and tragedies in the discovery of natural health care, will become familiar to the community at large.

Existing fractures in the health professions will be healed. Financial support through health-care providers and insurers will some day soon give Chiropractic it's rightful place, a place where all can access natural health care.

Healing takes place through non-linear

Clarity of purpose is communion with the soul. The voice inside becomes greater than the obstacles outside.

~Angelica E. Wagner

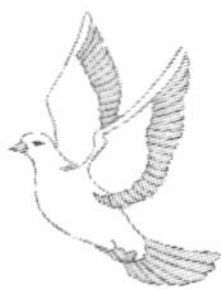

intention of thought and adjustment of the indicators of disease, through the hands and visualization of the healer.

By breaking out of patterns where we were previously stuck, our intellect finds reliable, systematic ways to improve our life and our health. Our body finds its own path to healing. Only when there is openness and receptiveness in the nervous system can one also find receptiveness in the window of the human soul.

These old patterns, broken one at a time, open to the most appropriate path to freedom and occur at the most appropriate time. In every cycle in linear time, there are adjustments to new thoughts and better methods. These then transcend the old ways and create new processes. Just as the Chiropractic adjustment is the most effective process for healing interferences in the body, the most effective change in society will occur with inspiration rather than with force. Openness to change medical opinions will create a just, compassionate society through the realms of healing and in the unification of all health-care professionals.

Let "the innate power" adjust the body by giving it time and permission to find its own path. As a society breaking free from its own stuck patterns of guilt, anger, control or fear, indicators in the cycles of historical time shall also find Chiropractic as a path to wholeness in modern health care.

Transformation of the Universe

For those of us who have experienced miracles, we see them as a liberating, enhancing, transforming intervention of God. Individuals liberated from illness and from disease are restored not only to themselves, but to their relationships with others. They are enabled to begin life anew, to choose new directions and new beginnings. Miracles urge us not to base our lives on the security of physical determinism, but rather on the mystery of God who creates and restores life. There is a higher power within us and around us that makes all things possible and all miracles real.

Miracles, therefore, not only bring saving grace to your life, but transform and enhance your life as expressions of glory and light. Miracles inspire the unconquerable spirit of

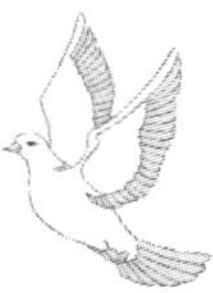

mankind to freedom and self-expression. Miracles speak to each of us in the very heart place of our deepest longings. The fullness of the expression of the soul is characterized by transformation, not just the transformation of the individual soul but the transformation of all humanity in the liberation of its talents and inherent power. The transformation of the universe lies in the transformation of each individual soul and the expression of that soul in its full potential. Are you expressing your full potential?

Miracles thus draw us toward the earth and at the same time detach us from it, calling on our senses to play in order to provide a new direction for the spirit. Miracles preserve the tension between time and eternity. Liberated spirit creates a new world order. It is the interplanetary light that dances between the stars to give us a glimpse of the future of undreamed wonders and raptures. In recognizing and honoring the raptures in our life, we liberate the spirit of total freedom and the endless possibilities of our own unlimited power.

Miracles, therefore, shed light on the inauguration of a new world order, a world of light and grace. This new world order is a reflection of the transformation that has begun in this current age. As we move into the new millennium, miracles will become commonplace. They will become daily occurrences to those who are aware of them and to those who seek them.

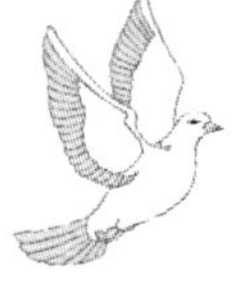

The purpose in each of our lives is to awaken mankind to total service and total love. Miracles always occur as an expression of love, love being the essence of all energy. Love is the unlimited power, infinite knowledge and absolute totality of all creative energy in its most perfect form. That is why the mystery of the miracle lies in messages of love toward each other and all humanity. Are you expressing love in order to create miracles?

If you're really ready for a miracle, learn to say "no" to those beliefs, actions and people that don't support your purpose. Learn to say "yes" to the truth of your internal being, the God-Self within you. You are ready for a miracle when your spirit is free and happy. You will have embraced love as the answer to the transformation of your own divinity. The essence and power of your immortal soul will emerge in its magnificent glory.

Remember, you are the miracle!

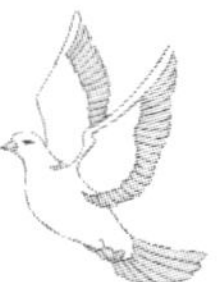

Are You Ready for... More Miracles?

Do you or someone you know have a story or article that you think should be shared with others to give hope or help inspire? If you do, please send it to me.

Miracleworks International Inc.
P.O. Box 53011
5100 Erin Mills Parkway
Mississauga Ontario
L6M 6C4
Fax (905) 812-7202
1-877-MIRICLE

I will make sure that you and the author are credited for the contribution. Thank you!

LECTURES, SEMINARS AND WORKSHOPS

You can also contact me at the above address for speaking engagements or for information about other books, audio tapes, workshops and training programs.

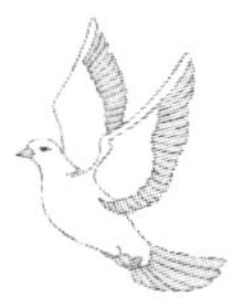

Are You Ready for a Miracle with Angels?

I have brought together a collection of stories about healing angels in order to honor life and the healing profession. These stories are a series of miracles – all true, all factual – that caused a life change for those who experienced them. Miracles have inspired, given purpose and direction

Don't miss reading this wonderful book – your life may never be the same again.

Yours with Success,
Angelica Wagner

ORDER FORM

Name: ____________________

Address: ____________________

City: ____________________

Province/State: ____________________ Postal/Zip Code: ____________

Phone Number: ____________________ Facsimile Number: ____________

Please send me :

____________ copies of

Are You Ready for a Miracle? with ... Angels

@ $ 16.95 ea. Canadian
$ 14.95 ea. U.S.

SUBTOTAL ____________

GST ____________

PST ____________

TOTAL ____________

METHOD OF PAYMENT

☐ Cheque enclosed
☐ Mastercard / Visa

____
Credit Card Number:

____
Expiry Date

____
Signature

MAIL TO: **MIRACLEWORKS INTERNATIONAL INC.**
P.O. Box 53011, 5100 Erin Mills Parkway, Mississauga, ON L6M 6C4
Telephone: 1-877-MIRICLE
Facsimile: 1-905-812-7202

Change has ALWAYS brought opportunity for those who have the courage to act.

Many of those who have purchased "Secrets of Success" have already achieved their desired goals with outstanding and extraordinary results … for them, business is booming!

Let me help you turn fear into courage as you apply the principles of proven success. Why not start now, and watch your business take off! Since you are already doing what you love to do, "Secrets of Success in Real Estate Excellence" will only further inspire you to do it in the BEST ways possible. Make the choice NOW for your future.

Yours with Success,

Angelica Wagner

ORDER FORM

Name: ____________________

Address: ____________________

City: ____________________

Province/State: ____________________ Postal/Zip Code: ____________

Phone Number: ____________________ Facsimile Number: ____________

Secrets of Success Workbook	$29.95
Secrets of Success Tapes Series	
(East)	$159.00
(West)	$159.00
Courage Tape	$10.00
Purchase any one tape and book	$179.00
Purchase any two tapes and book	$300.00

SUBTOTAL ____________

GST ____________

PST ____________

TOTAL ____________

METHOD OF PAYMENT

☐ Cheque enclosed

☐ Mastercard / Visa

____
Credit Card Number:

____
Expiry Date

____
Signature

MAIL TO: **MIRACLEWORKS INTERNATIONAL INC.**
P.O. Box 53011, 5100 Erin Mills Parkway, Mississauga, ON L6M 6C4
Telephone: 1-877-MIRICLE
Facsimile: 1-905-812-7202

An extensive library of Angelica Wagner's ongoing live lectures are available on audio and visual cassette and may be ordered by calling

1-877-MIRICLE

in Canada and U.S.A.